Leonard of Bertapaglia: On Nerve Injuries and Skull Fractures

Number 52

The History of Medicine Series
Issued under the Auspices of
the Library of
The New York Academy of Medicine

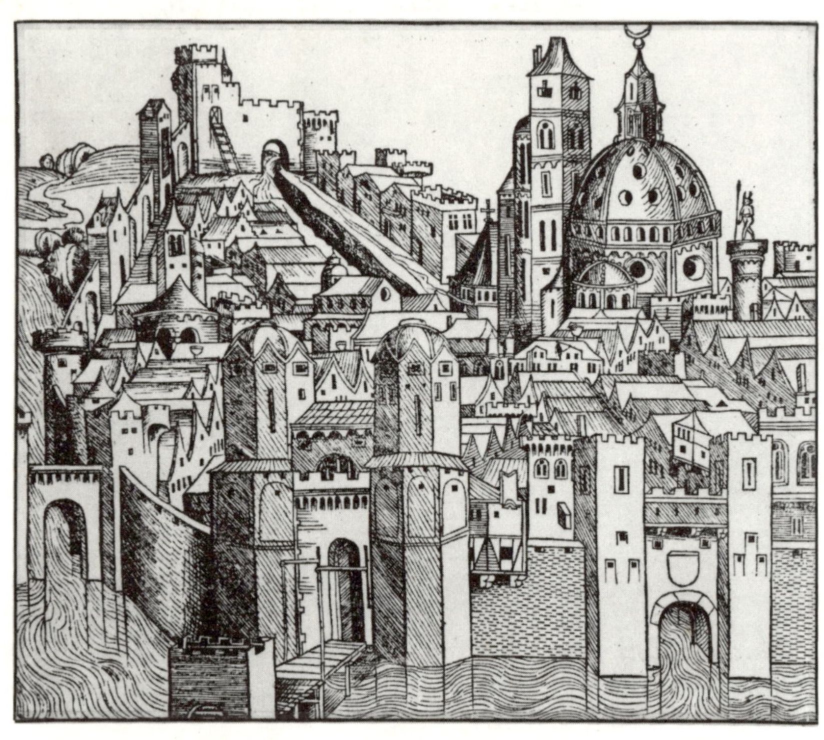

"Fair Padua. Nursery of arts." ... *Shakespeare. (Reproduced with permission, Schedel, Hartmann, [Liber chronicarum], Nuremberg, 1943, folio 44 verso ["Fair Padua"]; Rare Book and Manuscripts Division, The New York Public Library, Astor, Lenox and Tilden Foundations.)*

Leonard of Bertapaglia: On Nerve Injuries and Skull Fractures

Translated, with an Introduction and Commentary

by

Jules C. Ladenheim, M.D.

Foreword by

Professor Sir Sydney Sunderland
University of Melbourne

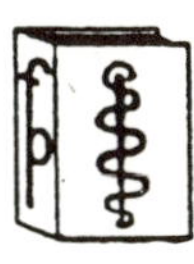

Futura Publishing Company, Inc.
Mount Kisco, New York
1989

Library of Congress Cataloging-in-Publication Data

Bertapaglia, Leonardo, ca. 1380–1463.
[Chirurgica. English. Selections]
Leonard of Bertapalgia : on nerve injuries and skull fractures / translated, with an introduction and commentary, by Jules C. Ladenheim ; foreword by Sir Sydney Sunderland.
p. cm. — (History of medicine series ; no. 52)
Translation of two chapters of: Chirurgica.
Bibliography: p.
ISBN 0-87993-326-7
1. Neurosurgery—Early works to 1800. I. Ladenheim, Jules C. (Jules Calvin), 1923– . II. Title. III. Series.
[DNLM: WZ 290 B536c]
RD593.B472513 1988
617′.48—dc19
DNLM/DLC 88-6995
for Library of Congress CIP

Published by
Futura Publishing Company, Inc.
295 Main Street, P.O. Box 330
Mount Kisco, New York 10549

LC# 88-6995
ISBN: 0-87993-326-7

TO
FRED LADENHEIM
1962–1982

*"Bleib' du im ew'gen Leben
Mein guter Kamerad..."*

Table of Contents

Foreword ix
Preface xi
Introduction xiii

I
Leonard of Bertapaglia:
Tractatus de Solutione Continuitatis Nervorum
On Injuries to Nerves
2

II
Commentary on Leonard of Bertapaglia's
On Injuries to Nerves
41

III
Leonard of Bertapaglia:
Capitulum de Fractura Cranei
On Skull Fractures
50

IV
Commentary on Leonard of Bertapaglia's
On Skull Fractures
109

V
Textual Criticism
129

VI
Pharmacopoeia
139

Foreword

The history of medicine is a long, complicated, and tortuous story which is incomplete in many respects. Quite rightly the subject continues to receive attention and any effort to rescue and preserve from obscurity something which is part of our heritage, no matter how small and seemingly unimportant, is a worthy undertaking and one that should be encouraged and supported.

It is, therefore, a pleasure to write this foreword to Dr. Ladenheim's contribution to this subject in the form of a translation of two chapters from Leonard of Bertapaglia's *Chirurgica*, one on "Nerves" and the other on "Skull Fractures," with appropriate commentaries on each. This is a well-researched and well-documented study of one of the prominent, but neglected and therefore lesser known, surgical figures of the period between the closing days of the Middle Ages and the dawn of the Renaissance. As such, the translation brings to our notice an interesting and readable account of surgical practice in the first half of the fifteenth century, an account which has the added attraction of giving special emphasis, for the first time, to nerve injuries and skull fractures, thereby providing an important work of reference for those with a particular interest in the origins of neurosurgery.

The fifteenth century is a period in the history of medicine which has attracted little attention, and about which little has been written, largely because it became completely overshadowed by interest in the times of Guy de Chauliac, the most celebrated authority on surgery in the fourteenth century, and subsequently, in the sixteenth century, by the exploits of the great Ambroise Paré and the genius of Vesalius, with his tradition-shattering observations which so dramatically broke new ground and established the foundation of scientific medicine.

Though a careful perusal of the chapters on nerves and skull fractures reveals little that was new or original, this should not be surprising, for this was a time when surgeons and physicians were practicing within constraints imposed not only by an uncritical

adherence to traditions and conventions handed down from the writings of Galen and Avicenna, but also by the authority of the Church, an authority which demanded unquestioned obedience to dogma, faith, and mysticism. Such an environment was not conducive to innovation and change, with the result that this became a colorless and lack-luster period of medical history in comparison with what had gone before and what was to follow.

The essential value of Leonard's writings lies in the fact that they provide an informative record of the "state of the art" in the surgical arena of the fifteenth century. Looked at in this light, he fulfills the important role of the conscientious custodian and disseminator of an established body of knowledge at a time when there was always the grave risk that information could become entirely lost because of increasing ignorance, neglect, and disuse.

Though Leonard's claims to lasting recognition may not be as strong as those of some of his predecessors, his writings leave no doubt that he was a thoughful and astute observer, mindful of maintaining and extending the quality of surgical practice at that time, and one of the most sought after, professionally competent, and successful surgical teachers and practitioners of his day. And despite the thought-crippling conventions of that period, he was getting close to the Renaissance attitude and spirit when he wrote: "Trust incompletely anything cited by authority unless it can be explained by experiment or by reason." He certainly deserves resurrecting and the author is to be congratulated on having undertaken, and successfully completed, this historical offering which should do much to establish Leonard's rightful place in the early annals of surgical history. This has been a painstaking assignment of immense labor, and we are indebted to Dr. Ladenheim for having carried so difficult a task to so admirable a conclusion.

Sir Sydney Sunderland
Professor Emeritus of Experimental Neurology
University of Melbourne
Melbourne, Australia

Preface

My attention was first directed to the *Cyrurgia* of Leonard by the late Professor Lynn Thorndike. This work continues the study undertaken at his suggestion. During my preparations, I have used the facilities of the Rare Book Room of the New York Academy of Medicine, the Biblioteca Riccardiana of Florence, the Royal Caroline Institute of Stockholm, and the New Jersey College of Medicine and Dentistry. I acknowledge with gratitude the courtesies shown me by the staffs. Mrs. Inge DuPont was especially helpful. My dear wife, Janet, assisted with the technical chores and revived my flagging initiative. To my secretaries, Mrs. Frances Shaw and Mrs. Jean Ganley, who added additional burdens to their work, I express my thanks.

Dr. Harold Fruchtbaum was most generous in reading the manuscript. To Professor Richard Carrubba, I express profound thanks for his enormous help and the patience shown my shortcomings. Lastly, and above all, Dr. William D. Sharpe refloated the grounded enterprise. His scholarly perceptions, treasured assistance, kindness, and generous encouragement continue to inspire me.

What errors and misinterpretations remain are my own.

Jules C. Ladenheim

Introduction

In the closing decade of the fifteenth century, an enterprising Venetian publisher prepared an anthology of surgical texts, probably for the use of medical students and practitioners, selecting eight distinguished manuscripts from the literature of the preceding three centuries. The authors and the selections appearing in the first edition of 1497 were shuffled about[1] in subsequent editions but, in general, included the surgical treatises of Roland, Roger, Bruno da Longaburgo, Theodoricus, Lanfrancus, William of Saliceto, Guy de Chauliac, and Leonard of Bertapaglia. This collection, later known as the *Collectio Chirurgia Veneta*, acquired great popularity during the following five decades and was reprinted in several editions. The contributions of the men contained in the collection stand as landmarks in the history of medicine.

Leonard of Bertapaglia alone has suffered from the vicissitudes of time. Although chosen to represent the fifteenth century surgeon in this distinguished surgical anthology, he lost his attraction during the centuries which followed.[2] He is mentioned in the *Historia Chirurgiae Antiqua*[3] (1713) as having flourished around 1520 and having been published with Roland, etc. The *Bibliotheca Chirurgica*[4] (1774) dismisses him as a "miserable superstitious astrologer... who, neverthless, often dissected." His name is listed in the *Bibliotheca Chirurgica* of de Vigiliis[5] (1781), his printed editions noted and the caustic observation made *faere totus est in medicamenta.* Sprengel[6] (1805) confines his remarks chiefly to the fact that Ber-

[1]The composition of the 1497, 1498, 1499, 1513, 1519 and 1546 editions are analysed by Edouard Nicaise, *La Grande Chirurgie de Guy de Chauliac.* (Paris, 1890), p. 129.

[2]He is cited by Bartholomeo dal Sarasin (fl. 1474) for his treatment of wounds. See Thomas Herndon, "A note on medieval wound treatment," *J. Hist. Med. Allied Sci. 19:*215, 1964.

[3]Andrea Ottomaro Goelicke, *Historia Chirurgiae Antiqua.* (Halle, 1713), p. 104.

[4]Albert von Haller, *Bibliotheca Chirurgica.* (Basel, 1774), vol. 1, p. 164.

[5]Stephan Hieronymus von Creutzenfeld de Vigiliis, *Bibliotheca Chirurgica.* (Vienna, 1781), vol. 1, p. 3.

[6]Kurt Sprengel, *Geschichte der Chirurgie.* (Halle, 1805), p. 15.

tapaglia devised thirty local applications for the cure of skull fractures.

Nor has criticism been more favorable in modern times. Gurlt[7] accords him less attention than any of the other authors found in the *Collectio* but his remarks are, nevertheless, of assistance. Castiglioni[8] records that he was "professor at Padua, published a *Recollecta super quartum Avicennae*, a book full of astrology and Arabian polypharmacy." Daremberg[9] is more charitable. He states that he "held on high the character and obligations of the true surgeon."

Of the early history of Leonard of Bertapaglia (variously spelled Bertapalia, Berti palia, Bertepaglia, Bertapalia, Berutapalia and Predapalia)[10] not much is known. His father was Bartholomew Bufo of Bertapaglia,[11] familiarily described as poor but honest.[12] Eloy[13] says that he was born in 1380 but cites no reference. However, since a medical student could not enroll before his twentieth birthday and since Gloria[11] states, from the records, that Leonard enrolled at Padua in 1400, one might surmise that the birthdate given by Eloy is not far from the mark. Tossoni[14] says he enrolled in 1402.

Padua[15] is close by the town of Bertapaglia, so it is not unexpected that the young student was drawn there. Founded in 1221[16]

---

[7]Ernest Julius Gurlt, *Geschichte der Chirurgie*. (Berlin, 1889), vol. 1, pp. 858–865.

[8]Arturo Castiglioni, *A History of Medicine*. (New York, 1941), p. 371.

[9]Charles Victor Daremberg, *Histoire des Sciences médicales*. (Paris, 1870), vol. 1, pp. lxxix, 317.

[10]Some of the variants in spelling are given in *La Grande Encyclopédie* (Paris, 1886), vol. 6, p. 433.

[11]A. Gloria, *Monumenta della Universita di Padova, 1318–1405*. (Padua, 1888), vol. 1, p. 444; vol. 2, p. 373. Quoted from Lynn Thorndike, *Science and Thought in the Fifteenth Century*. (New York and London, 1963), p. 62, and reverified for me by the library authorities of the University of Padua.

[12]Antoine Portal, *Histoire de l'anatomie et de la chirurgie*. (Paris, 1770), vol. 1, p. 238.

[13]Nicholas François Joseph Eloy, *Dictionnaire historique de la Médecine*. (Liege and Frankfurt, 1755), vol. 1, p. 150. That Leonard was a student duly enrolled can be verified from Gloria, reference 11 above.

[14]Pietro Tossoni, *Della Anatomia degli Antichii della Scuola anatomica Padovana: Memorie*. (Padua, 1844), p. 63.

[15]Lynn Thorndike, *Science and Thought in the Fifteenth Century*. (New York and London, 1963), p. 60. Professor Thorndike was fond of relating an accounting of his adventures in an inn in the town of Bertapaglia.

[16]Adolphe Pierre Burggraeve, *Précis de l'Histoire de l'anatomie*. (Gand, 1840), pp. 46, 51.

or 1222[17,18] in the aftermath of the Bolognese Forli[19] war, the university had become the great center of Averroistic tradition.[20] Its fame was at its zenith during the 15th century and its glory continued throughout Leonard's lifetime until eclipsed by the Turkish wars and the circumnavigation of the Cape of Good Hope.

The course in medicine required a minimum of four years with allowance for previous study in the arts[21], but more often it took longer. In addition to the habitation prerequisites, the bachelor's degree[22] required a public lecture on a chosen medical subject, as well as a disputation or two responses.[23] Graduation was not essential for the practice of medicine. Many students quit the university, early confident of a license to practice medicine from some local authority.[24] For those who sought an academic license, many universities required that the candidate study under supervision.[25,26] This Leonard did, for he alludes with reverence to his preceptors Lucca[27] and Betinus de Rabis.[28] We are told that Leonard also studied in Rome and Verona during his early training. Like many young physicians since the time of Galen,[29] Leonard sought to broaden his knowledge by travel. He tells us that he journeyed abroad in the service of the Venetian government, visiting the cities of Mecca and Alexandria,[30] where he treated a

---

[17]Thomas Louth, *Histoire de l'anatomie.* (Strasburg, 1815), p. 294.

[18]Pietro Capparoni, *Magistri Salernitani nondum cogniti.* (London, 1923), p. 4. [Research Studies in Medical History, No. 2]

[19]Hastings Rashdall, *Universities of Europe in the Middle Ages.* (Oxford, 1895), vol. 2, p. 11.

[20]John Herman Randall, Jr., *The School of Padua and the Emergence of Modern Science.* (Padua, 1961), p. 18.

[21]Theodor Puschmann, *A History of Medical Education*, Trans. E. H. Hare. (London, 1891), p. 261.

[22]Eileen Roach Cunningham, "Development of Medical Education and Schools of Medicine." *Ann. Med. Hist., N.S.* 7:223, 1935.

[23]For the curriculum and requirements for licensure, see Lynn Thorndike, *University Records and Life in the Middle Ages.* (New York, 1944), p. 321.

[24]Edouard Nicaise, *La Grande Chirurgie de Guy de Chauliac.* (Paris, 1890), p. li.

[25]Lynn Thorndike, ref. 23, p. 321, quotes Fournier.

[26]Rashdall, *op. cit.*, vol. 1, p. 242.

[27]Tr. II, Cap. 9; Tr. V, Cap. 1; Tr. II, Cap. 60.

[28]*Tr. de Vulneribus*, Cap. 9; *Tr. de Aegritudinibus ossium*, Cap. 5.

[29]M. Peynilke, *Histoire de la Chirurgie.* (Paris, 1780), vol. 2, pp. 533, 544, quoting Galen on travel as a necessity for physicians; Galen, *De compositione medicamentorum* 3.2.

[30]*De Fractura Cranei*, cap. 1 (MS).

Venetian nobleman for formica miliaris (punctuate rash).[31] Although he states he did this while on government mission, our suspicion is that he made the trip as a ship's doctor.

This journey to Mecca (more likely to Jiddah, the port) is the earliest reported visit to the Holy City by a Western Christian but it is quite probable that Venetian merchants had long been established in the Jiddah trade and had been practicing their calling for a century before the "discovery" of Mecca by John Cabot (between 1584–90), Piedro de Cavilhao (1494) and Lodovico Varthema (1503).

The *galere da mercato* on which we may presume Leonard sailed was probably of several hundred tons burden, armed with archers, soldiers and cannon,[32] and bound in convoy by way of Rhodes[33] for Alexandria, where it arrived after a journey of 1–2 weeks. From a staging area 10 miles outside of Alexandria, enormous caravans departed after Ramadan, travelling across the Isthmus of Suez and along the eastern shore of Red Sea. These self-sufficient and well-defended caravans, composed of tens of thousands of merchants and pilgrims and a corresponding number of mules and camels, arrived after 40 days, in Jiddah.[34] There, negotiations would commence for the spices, pearls, silk, and perfumes so adored by the West.

Leonard received his license[35] in medicine on January 21, 1412, following private and public examinations. This license legitimized the use of the title of *Magister*, or Master, although the title was informally appropriated by anyone enrolled in the course of medicine.[36] He began practice in the city of Padua, a bold undertaking for the young graduate. Some years later, Leonard was invited to lecture at the university, but, not having a doctorate, he was assigned to so-called extraordinary subjects.[37] The ordinary lec-

---

[31]*Tr. de Apostematibus*, Cap. 3, 5.

[32]Luzzatto, Gino, An Economic History of Italy (London, 1961), p. 87.

[33]Pierre Belon, Les observations de plusieurs singularités et choses memorable trouvée in Grèce, Asie, Judée, Egypte, Arabie et autres pays estranges, Paris, 1553. Quoted from Pernand Braudel, *The Mediterranean* (New York, 1966) Vol. I, p. 363.

[34]Braudel, *ibid*, p. 181.

[35]G. Zonta and J. Brotto, *Acta graduum academicorum Gymnasii Patavini.* (Padua, 1922), p. 230.

[36]Pushmann, ref. 21, p. 262; Rashdall, *op. cit.*, vol. 1, p. 199.

[37]Rashdall, *op. cit.*, vol. 2, p. 11.

tures, lasting one and one-half hours, were given in the morning by doctors. The extraordinary lectures were given by licentiates for two hours in the afternoon.[38] Both categories of instructors were elected or appointed yearly,[39] and both were accorded the title of "professor."

The subject assigned to Leonard was a commentary on the fourth *Canon of Avicenna*.[40] The system of this Arab physician had been known to the Latin medical literature since the twelfth century through the translation of Gerald of Cremona.[41] Leonard probably began his lectures in 1417, and in accordance with the university requirements submitted a copy (exemplar) to the stationeries of the university before each term. This exemplar in turn was copied and lent out by stationeries to the students for a sum prescribed by university statute. About sixteen manuscripts[40] have survived, attesting to the demand. Leonard is said to have attracted many students to his lectures.[41] At the time his course was first offered, he is known to have had a 11 year old son, Fabricius.[42] Leonard acquired a distinguished reputation in Padua and a large practice in nearby Venice,[43] Padua then being a Latin Quarter for the mighty mistress of the Adriatic.[44] He acquired great wealth, of which he gave liberally to the construction of public buildings in Padua and its environs.[45] At the time of his death, he lived in the Via Galilei, then the Pozzo del Campioni, which one learns from the *Archivi di Stato de Padova*.[46]

Cadaver dissection is said to have been formally inaugurated in Padua in 1429, although prior to that date necropsies had been performed for medico-legal purposes,[47] and of course, animal dis-

---

[38]Thorndike, ref. 23, p. 142, quotes Osler Library MS. 7554, ff. 19v, 21v-22r.

[39]Rashdall, *op. cit.,* vol. 1, pp. 248, 191.

[40]Judging from the curriculum at Bologna given in Thorndike, ref. 23, p. 278, the canon was an "extraordinary" subject given in the first year of medical study. Lynn Thorndike, "Another Manuscript of Leonard of Bertapaglia and John de Tracia." *Bull. Inst. Hist. Med. 4:*257–260, 1936.

[41]George Washington Corner, *Anatomical Texts of the Earlier Middle Ages.* (Washington, 1927), p. 27; *Nouvelle Biographie Générale* (Paris, 1852), vol. 5, p. 690.

[42]*De Fractura Cranei*, cap. 1 (MS).

[43]Salvatore de Renzi, *Storia della Medicina in Italia.* (Naples, 1845), p. 441; Papadopoli, *Historia Gymnasii Patavini.* (Venice, 1726), p. 285.

[44]Ernest Renan, quoted in Rashdall, *op. cit.,* vol. 2, p. 11.

[45]Tossoni, *op. cit.,* p. 63.

[46]Arch. di Stato di Padova, Estimo Anno 1418, Tome 22, No. 34.

[47]Nicaise, ref. 1, p. liii.

section had been permitted.[49] One is uneasy with this late date for dissection (1429)[50] because as early as 1405, Bologna is known to have authorized dissection. It seems curious, if not improbable, that Padua's celebrated medical faculty would have waited a quarter of a century to follow suit. At any rate, on February 8, 1429, Leonard is known to have given a course of surgery conjointly with Hugh of Siena, dissecting an executed murderer from Bergamo. "I assisted with Master Leonard in charge of the course of surgery," writes a copyist in the *De Annectotis.*[51] Leonard was no mere spectator but drew on anatomic dissection to aid his surgical instruction. He is known to have been present at other dissections in 1439 and 1440,[52] but extant records of his attendance pale before those of Montagnana[53] who is reported to have been present at no fewer than fourteen dissections.

Alas, Leonard's success won for him not only fame but bitter hostility as well. A morsel of evil gossip is preserved by the copyist of the Florentine manuscript of 1424, who records: "Here follows the surgery of Master Leonard of Bertapalia who has not received his degree [i.e., doctorate] in surgery because of the hostility.[54] Leonard's tactlessness, or the envy engendered by a large and successful surgical practice, evidently raised the hackles of his colleagues. We have a record in the same year (1424) of a petition forwarded by several members of the faculty to the Doge of Venice, to the effect that "It has recently been brought to our hearing that some of our doctors teaching in the University of Padua very frequently with your permission, and possibly without it, leave Padua

---

[48]J. W. L. Gruender, *Geschichte der Chirurgie*, second ed. (Breslau, 1865), pp. 123, 137.

[49]In 1308, the Senate of Venice ordered one cadaver to be dissected each year; Benjamin Lee Gordon, *Medieval and Renaissance Medicine.* (New York, 1959), p. 421. I am aware that Padua did not come under Venetian rule until 1405. (See Randall, ref. 20, p. 26).

[50]Charles Joseph Singer, *The Evolution of Anatomy.* (London, 1925).

[51]"By the outstanding and singular doctor, Master Hugh of Siena, lecturer here in ordinary, in the morning in a house near St. Luke's in the Paduan territory, and I was present at it with Master Leonard, lecturer in surgery." Quoted from Thorndike, in the manuscript text of the *Cyrurgia*, p. 271, who obtained it from the 1546 edition. I have not used this edition, but the passage in the 1498 edition appears to be similar.

[52]Lynn Thorndike, ref. 15, p. 61.

[53]Heinrich Haeser, *Lehrbuch der Geschichte der Medizin.* (Jena, 1845), p. 220.

[54]Expletum et hoc opus compositum Padue Anno 1424 per excellentissimum cirurgie magistrum Leonardum de Bertapalea qui numquam volent graduari propter excusare vituperium multorum doctorum ignorantium; nam potius voluit esse bonus acutifer quam malus miles. Cod. Bisconiana 13, f. 68v.

for the purpose of transacting various business of their own, deserting their lectures with the greatest annoyance and embarrassment to their students...".[55] Leonard's name is conspicuously absent from the list of signers.

At any rate, the doctorate[56] was not conferred on Leonard until June 12, 1450, when he was granted the privilege of reading, interpreting, and disputing in surgery.[57] With the privilege of the doctorate went the right to give ordinary lectures, in contrast to the extraordinary lectures given by licentiates. Moreover, he was granted a stipend of about 100 *lire*[58] a year subject to annual renewal by the Tractatores Studei[59] and, of course, the privilege of wearing a cape of purple and miniver![60]

Leonard died on December 15, 1463, as documented from the record of the tax assessor[61] before whom Leonard's heirs appeared to probate his will.

During his lifetime Leonard wrote, in addition to the *Cyrurgia*, tractates entitled "Antidotes," "Solutions for Skin Diseases";[62] "The Judgment and Prognostications of Wounds", and "Medical and Astronomical Chapters". Another work, "Judgment of the Revolution," was discovered by Thorndike in the manuscript of the *Cyrurgia*.[62] It is not unlikely, recalling Scareoni's[63-65] assertion that in his

---

[55]Lynn Thorndike, ref. 23, pp. 201–202.

[56]For the doctoral requirement, see Thorndike, ref. 23, p. 384.

[57]"Licentiam legendi, glosandi, interpretandi, medendi et omnes actus cirogicales," *Acta gradum academicorum Gymnasii Patavini*, Arch. Ant. dell Univ. de Padova, Register of Examinations, Doctorate of the University, No. 310, 25. Thorndike states that this refers to another Leonard, but I respectfully disagree.

[58]Lynn Thorndike, ref. 23, p. 360, quotes Borsetti Ferranti Bolani, *Historia Almi Ferrariae Gymnasii*, 1735, vol. 1, pp. 93–96.

[59]Rashdall, *op. cit.*, vol. 2, p. 11.

[60]Rashdall, *op. cit.*, vol. 1, p. 197.

[61]"Heredi quondam maistro Leonardo de Bertepaia medego" presented their petition to the tax assessor (Arch. di Stato di Padova, Estimo Anno 1418, Tome 22, No. 44).

[62]*De aquis conficiendis ad pellendas aegritudines maxime idoneis; Receptae datae super tertiam, quartam et quintam fen quarto canonis Avicennae; Capitulum de judiciis vulnerum significantium mortem; Judicium revolutionis anni 1427; Tractatus medicus et astronomicus* (Riccardiana Library): *De antidotis*. Thorndike states that the *De antidotis* is a compilation, probably made by a student, of Leonard's cures and miscellanea (See ref. 11, p. 68). With regard to the *Capitulum de judiciis vulnerum significantium mortem*, this was catalogued as a separate tractate by Valentinelli (1872, V.100), but challenged by Thorndike (ref. 11, p. 67) because no *explicit* separates it from the *Cyrurgia* in the Vatican MS.

[63]Jacobo Facciolati, *Fasti Gymnasii Patavini Patavii.* (Padua, 1957), p. 139.

[64]Scardeonius, *De Antiquitatibus Urbis Patavii*, vol. 2.ix, p. 209, quoted by Facciolati, ref. 63, and by Giovanni Maria Mazzuchelli, *Gli Scrittori d'Italia.* (Brescia, 1760), vol. 2, part 2, p. 1032.

[65]Zedler, *Grosses Universal Lexicon* (Leon, 1666), quotes Scardeonius.

lifetime Leonard wrote much and that other manuscripts await discovery.

To compare manuscript with incunabula is at once intriguing and informative. The editor of the incunable fashioned his edition for the contemporary medical market. He found in the seventy-year-old manuscript an account which was "quaint, garrulous and rather breathless, somewhat deficient in point of grammatical corrections and elegance."[66] Such literary defects, tolerated 67 years earlier when the manuscript first saw light, were unacceptable to an editor constricted by the enormous changes in literary standards brought about by printing.

With this in mind, the editor prepared a careful revision of the text. A passage describing a successful operation was deleted. The case history of a knife wound is omitted, as well as other passages describing contemporary medical practice. Language and grammar were polished, rubrics altered, and composition "enlivened" with all the literary subtleties.

What emerges is a masterful job of polishing, performed with fidelity to and respect for the original manuscript. This surely made the study of Leonard considerably more pleasant and convenient for medical studies of the late fifteenth century.

Unfortunately, the deletions expurgated from the printed editions are the very things of interest today to students of the history of medicine, and by his activity the editor has denied us insight into some interesting facets of Leonard's practice. Thanks to the scholarly efforts of the late Professor Thorndike, the matter has again been brought under scholarly scrutiny.

Leonard apparently had special instruction in neurosurgery. He devoted one-third of his book on surgery to the study of the then treatable illnesses of the nervous system, a far greater proportion than any of his predecessors. In succeeding centuries he is cited for his surgery on the nervous system, although his praise is neither uniform nor profuse. De Renzi[67] declares "the surgical care especially is simple and good and differs as relating to treatment of lesions of the nerves and fractures of the skull." Dezeimeris[68] states

---

[66]Thorndike, ref. 11, p. 70.

[67]De Renzi, ref. 43, vol. 2, p. 441.

[68]Jean-Eugène Dezeimeris, *Dictionnaire historique de la Médecine ancienne et moderne.* (Paris, 1828), vol. 1, p. 366.

that he completely neglected surgical operations and partook entirely of the existing judgments. Leonard is praised by Bernstein[69] (1822) for his treatment of skull fractures. To Grunder[70] he is *sehr naiv.* Billroth and Lueck[71] have scant mention of him.

Leonard's star was briefly rekindled by the research of Malgaigne[72] who credits Leonard with reintroduction of the crown trepan. This round drill, known to Hippocrates, had passed into oblivion by the time of Galen and remained forgotten during the middle ages. Malgaigne, moreover, focused attention on Leonard's contribution to vascular surgery. Leonard is said to have introduced the suture-ligature, whereby bleeding can be arrested by passing a suture through the blood vessel before it is tied,[73,74] thus assuring that the ligature will not later slip off. This principle of transfixion is an important advance over the practice of simple ligation popularized by Albucas[75] and Galen.[76]

For the reasons given above, I feel justified in proposing reexamination of the text of Leonard's *Chirurgica*. I have limited this survey to the sections dealing with neurological illnesses. These I have collated, translated, and interpreted in keeping with Professor Thorndike's statement, "A new edition of his text, based on manuscripts... would seem to be highly desirable."[77]

---

[69]Johan Gottlieb Bernstein, *Geschichte der Chirurgie.* (Leipzig, 1822), part 1, p. 138.

[70]J. W. L. Grunder, ref. 48, p. 137.

[71]Theodor Billroth and A. Luecke, *Uebersicht der Geschichte der Chirurgie und des Chirurgischen Standes.* (Stuttgart, 1879), vol. 1, p. 23.

[72]Joseph François Malgaigne, *Oeuvres complètes* d'Ambroise Pare. (Paris, 1840), pp. lxxxii-lxxxiii. I have since had the pleasure of examining the excellent translation by W. B. Hamby (University of Oklahoma Press).

[73]Et postea liga ipsam cum filo lineo ut melium et tenacius teneatur perfora dictam venam cum acu et cum filo circumcirc. Gurlt, *op. cit.,* vol. 1, p. 859.

[74]Samuel Clark Harvey, *History of Hemostasis.* (New York, 1929), p. 37.

[75]Amin Khairallah, "Arabic Contributions to Anatomy and Surgery." *Ann. Med. Hist., Third Ser. 4:*409, 1942.

[76]David Hosack, *Observations on the Surgery of the Ancients.* (New York, 1813), p. 21.

[77]Lynn Thorndike, "The Manuscript Text of Cyrurgia of Leonard of Bertipaglia." *Isis 1:*264-284, 1926.

Note

Throughout the texts, material unique to the manuscript is given in italics, while incunabular variants are enclosed within parentheses.

I

Leonard of Bertapaglia: Tractatus de Solutione Continuitatis Nervorum

I

[61r] (Tractatus IIII.) *Incipit tractatus* de solutione *continuitatis* (continui) nervorum. (De egritudinibus nervorum spectantibus ad cyrurgicum in universali. Capitulum Unum.)

Pretiosum (Preciosum) organum organorum in *cuis* (quo) est sensus manifestus, et motus voluntarius et naturalis; habet principium et originem immediate, et hoc secundum medicos, a cerebro ex parte septum *neruorum paria* (parium nervorum), que orta sunt *sub* (a) medio commissure *coronali* (coronalis); vel orta sunt ab ipso mediante nucha; que est tanquam vicarius cerebri ex parte aliorum nervorum descendentium ab hoc planta inferius natura magisteria cum *pervenit* (pervenerit) ei contrarietas *et rebellio,* accidunt ex vulneribus vehementes lesiones atque dolores et in to[l]lerabiles, et alia mala sicut spasmus *et* permixtio rationis stupor paralesis deinde mors.

Dispositiones que *valde* apte sunt consequi ad vulnera nervorum sunt dolor *febris* (febres), et apostemata sitis, et vigilie, et disiccatio lingue. Similiter hec eadem dispositio accidit in vulneribus chordarum *ac* (et) lacertorum et maxime in capitibus ipsarum. Sed quando nervi, et c[h]orde, et mus*ch*uli, et ligamenta (sicut genu) apostemantur sepe propter nimiam eorum repletionem atque immoderata(m) extensione(m) (spasmantur). Et si adveniat res putrefaciens, membrum corrumpitur; qualis est frigus quod festinat ad hoc (scilicet ad corruptionem), quia nervi creati sunt ex humiditate quam congelavit *et coagulavit* frigus. Omnis

I

Leonard of Bertapaglia: On Injuries to Nerves

[61r] Concerning the disruption of the continuity of nerves in general. Concerning nerve diseases of a surgical nature.

Chapter I

The most precious organ of all organs, wherein sensation is revealed as well as voluntary and involuntary movement, the nervous system, according to physicians, has its principle and direct origin in the cerebrum, where seven pairs of nerves emerge from the middle of the coronal commissure. The nerves also arise from the interposed brain stem, which is considered to be a proxy for the cerebrum. Thence, the nerves descend to the sole of the foot. Because of the strange, marvelous and occult qualities of its majestic nature, when a wound brings something untoward and rebellious into contact with the nerve, violent lesions, pain and unpleasant things ensue, as well as such harmful consequences as spasm, disorientation[1] (of reason), anesthesia,[2] paralysis and finally death.

The symptoms[3] which are likely sequelae of a nerve injury are pain, fever, pus, thirst, insomnia and a dry tongue. Similarly, these same symptoms occur in wounds of the sinews,[4] arms,[5] and especially with wounds of the head. When the nerves, sinews, muscles and ligaments (such as the knee) fester, they become spastic, be-

[1]permixtio rationis
[2]stupor
[3]dispositiones
[4]chordae
[5]lacerta

quidem putrefactio *occurrenti* (occurrens) nervo pervenit ex caliditate et humiditate immoderate ap[p]licata. Aqua quidem frigida ipsi nocet, ex parte spasmi, et calida ex hoc quod putrefacit. (Et optime nota) Dictum Galieni *quod* aqua (quidem) calida *est* mitigativa omnium dolorum preterquam in punctura nervorum non est ap[p]roximanda. Et similiter aliquod oleum est inconveniens, (et) *Similiter si illud est necessarium, et illud quod est calefactum* (si est necessarium tunc calefac ipsum) propter necessitatem sedandi dolorem. Aut convenit causa subtiliandi grossas medicinas, et ut eius virtus cito ad fundum *vulneris per*veniat, itaque quod resistant qualitati humectanti. Sed medicine pungitive, *sole autem* aliquando complent hanc *perfectionem* (intentionem). Ille qui vulneratus est in nervo et apostamatur, et est tarde resolutionis vel tarde maturationis et *successio ipsius* (susceptio illius) curationis est tarda, tunc ipsi nervi, quandoque ulcerantur, vel indurantur vel *infiltrantur in infiltratione qua vulnera* (infistulantur, qua infistulatione ulcera) redduntur tardioris, *resolutionis et* consolidationis, et tardioris maturationis.

(Tenere membrum is oleo calido sedat mirabiliter dolorem).

Vulnera que accidunt in nervis, aut est punctura aut (est) fissura longitudialis, aut fissura latitudinalis, aut *incisio* transversalis. Ex quibus quatuor omnibus aut sunt penetrantis ad utremque latus aut non. Aut nervus est cohopertus carne aut discoopertus ab ipsa. Et vulnera que fiunt in nervuo secundum longitudinem minus *iminet* (sunt) periculosa quam *cadentia* (accidentia) secundum latitudinem. Punctura vero sepe facit *accidere nervo vulnerato ad scissionem totalem* (nervuum venire ad totalem incisionem ipsius). Si volumus ipsum segregar(i)*e* a spasmo, [61ᵛ] et par hanc totalem incisionem perveniet quies, et seperabuntur accidentia mala quam vilus, sanus leditur *ex* (a) vicinitate incisi, et nocetur per ipsum, et inducit nocumentum cerebro, facient accidere spasmum et paralesim, et alia(s) *egritudines pravas* (accidentia mala).

Et Vulnera candentia in panniculis (ossium et aliis) sunt minus *periculosiora* (periculosa) eis que sunt *in cordis. Corde postea minus eis que sunt* in nervis, quoniam nervi sunt ad dandum sensum: c[h]orde vero in membro ad dandum motum. Et hoc sciri potest per testimonium anothomie *in corpore vivo et per discurssum rationis in ipso.* Nervus c[h]orda, panniculis, *ligamentum, atque* (et) cartilago differunt inter se *in duritie* (duricie) et *millitie* (mollicie) secundum magis et minus. Nam c[h]orda est dura valde, et non est panicularis in eius duri[c]*t*ie, et panniculus suffert suturam absque

cause of an excessive plethora[6] or excessive stretching. Then, if decaying elements[7] are present, the limb decomposes. One of the elements which accelerates corruption is cold. This is because nerves are created from the humors, which in turn can be congealed and coagulated by cold. All of the putrefying changes in the nerves are caused by the immoderate application of heat and moisture. Cold water harms the structure, inducing spasm, while warm water harms because it decays.[8] The best reference for this is found in the *Dicta* of Galen. Warm water assuages all pain but it should not be applied when the transected nerve has sustained a puncture injury. Oil, too, is unsuitable, but should its application be necessary, then warm the oil to soothe the pain. Warm oil is also useful for diluting thick medicines so that their beneficial powers may quickly reach the depths of the wound and combat the humoral qualities. Pungent medicines, too, sometimes accomplish this purpose. When the nerve is injured and pus forms, and the wound is late in resolving[9] or in maturing and the cure is slow, the nerves ulcerate, become indurated, or form fistulae. From these fistulae ulcers form which are slow to consolidate, resolve, and mature.[10]

(Placing the limb in warm oil diminishes the pain in miraculous fashion.)

Wounds which may befall nerves are as follows: punctures, fissures, both longitudinal and lateral, and transverse lacerations.[11] All these four injuries may or may not completely transect the nerve. The nerve may or may not be covered by flesh. Longitudinal nerve injuries are less dangerous than lateral nerve injuries. A puncture, moreover, often causes a complete nerve transection,[12] especially when we are trying to prevent spasm. [61^{v}] After complete transection, flaccid paralysis[13] results as well as other dire consequences. A covering of serosanguinous material[14] accumulates in the vicinity of the incision, which itself harms both wound and cerebrum, causing spasm, paralysis, and other untoward consequences.

[6]repletio
[7]res putrefaciens
[8]ex hoc quod putrefacit
[9]resolutio
[10]maturatio
[11]fissura
[12]incisio
[13]quies
[14]sanies

dolore *et nocumento*, sicut siphac quando suitur cum mirach. Et in vulneribus *ligamentarum talium* (ligamentalium) nascentibus ex osse, ad os non est de talibus accidentibus suspicandum, et suffert fortiorem curam. De nervo quo fuerit totaliter incisus sumus securi a spasmo; et si spasmus acciderit, (quod) timere debemus propter eorum contusionem et *de incisione partis eorum* (divisionem eius partium) in longitudine, et maxime corpori debili *et* existenti repleto.

II

Sequitur *Capitulum universale de Curatione Solutionis continuitatis vulnerum nervorum* (de solutione continuitatis nervorum in universali. Capitulum secundum.)

Et confirmatum est per sententiam *principis aboali* (Avicenni principis omnium medicorum) quod medicamen vulnerum nervorum debet esse calidum et siccum subtilium partium et equalis caliditatis *ita et* taliter, ut non mordic(a)et ipsum nervum, ad hoc, ut eius *exsiccatio* (exiccatio) fiat cum vehementia, et attractione multa, et non cum stipticitate superflua; *melius laudari et dici non posset.*

Porro omnis medicina in qua est caliditas subtilis cum *exsiccatione* (exiccatione) vehementi ad hoc ut prohibeat putrefactionem in nervuo non excusatur ab attractione multa. Et per hoc sepe cavendum est (de) *a* medicina stiptica, subtili, calida, et abstersiva, et maxima in principio ubi factam fuerit solutio continuitatis in nervos. Exemplus ut est si procederes cum ereysto, aut cum scoria, eris, et maxime in corpore existente repleto. In vulneribus quidem nervorum medicamen semper *tale medidicam* debet esse calefactionis temperate, et subtilis substantie, *et* (ut) in nervo melius cum sua virtute et forti exsiccatione penetret in ipso, et effectum inducat cum debita mensura et sine nocumento. Cum autem in nervo fuerit discooperatura, sufferre non potest aliquod acutum quia *est* sibi (infert) magnum nocumentum.

Wounds befalling the bony covering[15] and elsewhere are less dangerous than those of the sinews. Wounds to the sinew are not as dangerous as nerve wounds, for the nerves transmit sensation, while the sinews, of course, mediate movement in the extremity. This can be discerned through the testimony of living anatomy and from dialectics. Nerve, sinew, membrane, ligament, and cartilage differ among themselves, more or less, in respect to hardness and softness. The sinew is very hard, while the membrane less so, since the membranes can be sutured without pain and harm. Such is the case with the peritoneum[16] when the abdominal wall[17] is repaired. In wounds of the ligaments attached to bone, the bone is not liable to such consequences[18] and can tolerate a more stringent cure. Nerves that have been completely cut have the least likelihood of spasm. Should spasm occur, we must then consider contusion, partial longitudinal division, and especially plethora and debilitation.

Chapter II

The second general section concerns the cure of nerve lacerations.

In the opinion of Avicenna, foremost of all physicians, medication for nerve injuries should be warm, dry, fine in composition, and of measured heat, so as not to deaden[19] the nerve in question. This is the reason. Those medications which vigorously remove noxious material, draw, and are not too styptic, are the most praiseworthy.

Medicaments which are warm and have drawing properties such that they prevent putrefaction in the nerve can be relied upon to attract great quantities. Caution must be exercised that styptic medicines[20] be fine, warm and drawing,[21] especially when the nerve has been cut. An example would be if one were to begin treatment with hot copper[22] or with copper dross,[23] especially with

[15] pannicula
[16] siphac
[17] mirac
[18] accidentibus
[19] mordico
[20] stiptica
[21] abstertivim
[22] erysto
[23] scoria

Due intentiones in vulneribus nervorum, *medicus* in mente (medici) *semper* debent *habere* (occurrere). Prima ut non festinetur ad incarnationem, sed ut orificium vulneris stet apertum, ut ide materia expirare possit. Secunda intentio sit ut laboret (ut) iuxta suum posse, in removendo accentia que sequuntur, et sunt apta sequi ad talia vulnera; ut sunt dolor, spasmus, et apostemata, et hoc evaporando cum pannis calidis, et cum oleis circumcirca calefactis, et maxime cum *oleo onfrancino* (oleis onfrancinis), *quod* (que) *fit* (fiunt) ex olivis immaturis; quoniam in ipso est stipticitas, quedam cum adipibus; Iterum et fac quod illud sit actu calidum, *propter frigida*, et similiter seda apostemata (inquantum) potes (et). Dolor *non* (nullo modo) sedetur *nulla via mundi* cum aqua calida, sed cum oleo aliquo quod sit subtilium partium, et non habeat superfluam stipticitatem, *ymo* (immo) caliditatem non excedentem, quoniam calidum non superfluum prodest nervis. Frigidum vero *est valde inimicum* (mors). *Sepe vidi quod vulnus iam appropinquat* (Ipso sepissime vidi iam vulnera appropinquari) sanitati, et nocet ei(s) frigus *et accidetex illo* (ex quo accidit) maximus dolor et reddit *lesio* (lesionem), et *per* (propter) hoc est necessium ut succurratur statim ad sedandum dolorem cum oleis calefactis *embrocando* (imbrocando) *cum eis* et similter cum *butiro* (butyro) et sapa vini.

In nervo *vero* (autem) existenti discooperto cum incisione secundum longitudinem stude inquantum potes ad incarnandum et ad cooperiendum, et hoc *fieri* oportet cum medicamine et ligatura convenienti. Sed si nervus habeat vulnus in latitudine[m] sive vulnus existens in carne dimitendo [62^{r}] nervum, et si non suitur *tale* vulnus nervus non conglutinatur conglutioatione bona *tanquam bona secundum quod expedit.* Sed quando nervus ex toto non indicitur et timemus de spasmo et eius putrefactione*m* succure quantum est possibile cum medicinis removentibus ista. Sed si nervus fuerit cum puntura ne accidan*tur* accidentia mala *amplietur* illa punctura (scilicet incidendo totum nervuum) quoniam illud perducet fortasse ad putrefactionem, propter illud quod aggregatur de virulentia, et (de) putredine mala. (Nota.) Fuge *in* quantum potes aquam in vulneribus nervorum *approximate* quia corrumpit complexionem ipsius, ex parte superflue frigitatis, et ipsum putrefacit ex parte humiditatis, et per hoc oleum non est necessarium nisi calidum, et hoc per sedatione doloris, (quando aliter sedari non potest), et non labores in abluendo tale vulnus existens in nervo, neque cum oleo neque cum aqua; immo absterge humiditates cum pannis, aut coto

the body in a state of plethora. For nerve wounds one must insure that the medicines are moderately warm and thin in consistency so that their strength and drying properties can better reach the nerve, thereby promoting their benefits in the proper proportions and without causing harm. However, when the nerve is severed, it cannot tolerate anything sharp,[24] for this will cause great harm.

Concerning nerve wounds, the physician should remember two intentions. First, the wound should not be permitted to heal prematurely; rather, the wound orifice should always remain open to permit the discharge of material. Second, the physician should do his utmost to prevent such complications as pain, spasm and pus. This can be accomplished by drawing[25] with a hot eufranc oil[26] made from unripe olives, since it has styptic properties, and by the use of various fats. Prepare these things rather hot, to ease the pus as much as possible. Pain is in no way relieved by warm water, but by bland and moderately styptic medicines. Nor should heat be excessive. While withholding heat does not help the nerve, cold, so to speak, is death to that structure. I have often seen wounds nearly cured[27] harmed by cold, resulting in great pain and a recurrent lesion. Therefore, one must promptly relieve pain by applying[28] heated oil, together with butter and thick wine.

In nerves severed longitudinally, do your best to promote healing[29] and union.[30] This can be done with bindings[31] and appropriate medicines. If the nerve has a side-to-side injury or if the wound penetrates [62^r] the flesh and cuts the nerve, and this wound not be sutured, the nerve will not unite well, i.e., according to what is helpful. Further, when the nerve is incompletely cut and we fear spasm and putrefaction, we should do our best to remedy this with medicines. If the nerve has a puncture wound, beware lest a bad accident enlarge that puncture and cause a complete cut. This produces violent putrefaction which gathers slime and putrescence. Note: in nerve injuries, avoid water as much as possible for it cor-

---

[24]acutus
[25]evaporo
[26]pannis
[27]sanitus
[28]imbrocando
[29]ad incarnandum
[30]cooperiendum
[31]ligatura

quanto levius potes, et similiter non agas cum *acino cotto* (aceto) nisi fueris securus a nocumento humiditatis ipsius.

Sed quando in huiusmodi vulneribus fuerit punctura et discoopertura, et non cum apostema perveni ad localia medicamem. Nam tale medicamen oportet ut sit cum magna caliditate, et forti exsiccatione plusquam illud quod ponitur supra s[c]issura[m], quoniam via est parata ut medicamen penetret facilius ad egritudinem.

Dieta ergo in habentibus vulnera nervorum sit subtilis, et *sit* in ultimo subtilitatis. Nam cum in talibus vulneribus erit dolor qui facit accidere apostema similiter probe cibum subtilem et proprie quando vulnera sunt in latitudine, *uti flobothomia* (flobotomia) fortasse erit necesse, et *farmatia* (farmacia) et enemata, et alia divertentia. Comfortare membra propinqua vulneri cum unctionibus, sicut *in* ungere caput et collum et subasselas et inguina et spinam que *compatiuntur per cominitatem prestabitur vulneri per hoc magnum iuvamentum* (patiuntur membro leso et per hoc praestabitur magnum iuvamentum).

III

Sequitur capitulum de Glutino Albotim.

Glutinum (glutamen) albotim *vere* debemus intelligere *esse lacrimum* (de lachrymo) et non terbentinam ut affirmavit *dinus* (Dynus) sive oleum vicii quod (idem) est, de melioribus medicinis in vulneribus nervorum que in mundo *reperiri possit* (haberi possint). Sed loco ipsius *lacrimi* (lachrymi) utimur, *et hoc de* qui pro quo, et utimur terbentina et hoc in complexione infantium et in *mulieribus et in cuius complexio vehemens humiditatis* (vulneribus cuius complexio est vehementia humiditatis). Sed si *lacrimum* (lachrymum) esset durum, et siccum et antiquum, tunc incorpora ipsum cum pauco oleo rosato et melle rosato ut fluxibile et currens fiat. In corporibus *vero* (autem) siccis, et *in* cuius caro est dura oportet ut misceatur cum eo euforbium, quia antequam pervenita ad fundum vulneris iudica ut *remictatur* (remitatur) de eius caliditate et siccitate, et per hoc de ipso pone parum *vel* (et) multum secundum *quod complexionem* (calefactionem) corporis, et eius *calefactionem* (complexionem).

rupts the nerve's complexion[32] when it cools, and dampness causes putrefaction. For this very reason, unless oil be warm, it should not be applied, except to soothe pain, which cannot otherwise be soothed. Do not irrigate[33] nerve wounds with oil or water, but rather remove[34] the humidity gently with a dressing or a cotton[35] and avoid vinegar[36] unless you are safe from the danger of humidity.

When wound punctures and nerve cuts[37] occur in the absence of pus, the medicine must be able to reach the area. Such medicines must generate great heat and have drawing properties greater than those used above a laceration,[38] for way must be made for the medicine to penetrate easily to the morbid process.[39]

The diet for those who have nerve wounds should be bland, in fact, exceedingly bland.[40] In such wounds, when pain ensues causing the formation of pus, try a bland diet. Where a transverse nerve wound has occurred, a vigorous phlebotomy[41] may be necessary, along with drugs,[42] enemata, etc. Soothe the injured area with unctions, applying them to the head, neck, axilla,[43] groin,[44] and spine. These regions, as well as the nerve, are in pain and, when anointed, great relief is afforded the wound.

Chapter III

A section concerning white glue.

With regard to the saps,[45] we ought to use white glue, rather than turpentine, as Dynus observes, or the viscid oils, which are the same. It is the best medicine for nerve wounds. In place of saps,

[32]complexio
[33]abluendo
[34]abstergero
[35]coto
[36]aceto
[37]discoopertus
[38]scissura
[39]aegritudinem
[40]subtilis
[41]flebotomia
[42]farmacia
[43]subassaelas
[44]inguina
[45]lacrymo

Loco vero euforbii administra lac titimali, *laureola* (laureole),*exsula anabula* (exula) de qua fit scamonea, quoniam ista sunt mirabilia sed ea que sunt debiliora his sunt sicut *assa* (rasa) serapinum, opponacus, baurac, *et* spuma maris, et sulfur calefac(i)um cum oleo olive, et omne medicam[en] quod est attractivum, *humiditatum* (humectativum) ad exteriora, sicut fermentum et similia, (et in eo) vidi magnum iuvamentum, quam attrahit *ex* (a) profundo *actractione* (attractione) bona. Terbentina *vero est melior res* (autem est de melioribus) cum *qua incipit* (quibus incipimus).

Glutinum species (species glutini) que convenire possunt in vulneribus nervorum sunt *otto* (octo). *Prima raxa* (primo rasa) pini. Secunda (Secundo) rasa *abieti* (abici). *Tertia* (tertio) *raxa* (rasa) *pencem* (penzeni). *Quatro* (Alia) *raxa* (rasa) *arda* que colofonie dicitur. *Sexta* (Alia) *raxa* (rasa) alba orta *est* a piceo albo, et dicitur terventina. *Septima* (Alia) *raxa* (Rasa) me*l*lina. *Octa* (Alia) rasa *oleginea* (oleagina), (et dicitur orta ab arbore vicii *et* (ut) dicitur *lacrimum* (lachrymum). Et omnes *este otto* (istas octo) species largo modo appellare possumus glutina. *Sed* (et) sepe ista abluimus quando volumus diminuere *earum* (eorum) acuitatem. Medicamen quod convenit in punctura nervorum propter eius stricturam debet esse maioris caliditatis et siccitatis cum subtiliori substantia, ut velocius penetret ad *fundum* (fondum) quam medicamen quod approximatur in incisione. Sed quando accidit putrefactio in talibus [62v] vulneribus laudatum est serapinum et farina orobi. Item *vinum* (coctum) sapa cum calamento, et oleo communi in forti dolore omnes *sapientis* (periti) medici concedunt.

Galienus studendum ut medicamen sit subtiliativum et temperatum in calore siccitatem prestans sine dolore. In principio si vulnus sit simplex utamur glutino albotim id est gummi abietis in quo dissolvatur pulveris lombricorum terrestrium exiccatorum in umbra, et actu ponatur calidum. Si vero vulnus sit co[n]positum sicciora conveniunt, et hoc magis et minus secundum complexionem et magnitudinem apostematis.)

(Temperate caliditatis est hoc. Rx: florum camomille, absinthii, pulegii ana M. i; farine fabarum, farine lupinorum ana unc. iiii; olei camomellini, olei sambucini ana unc. iiii; pulveris lumbricorum unc. ii; Fiat emplastrum, sed omnia decoquantur in lixivio, et sic canonice operando omnis dolor cessabit et habebis honorem.)

(Si vero fuerit spasmus in facie, tunc fiat inunctio in occipitio tunc ponatur desuper oleum quasi fervens oleum de euforbio, et

turpentine may be substituted when dealing with infant and female complexions and in wounds having an exceedingly humid complexion. Where the sap is firm, dry or old, admix a small amount of red oil and red honey to thin it out. Where the body is dry and the flesh[46] hard, it is best to mix euforbius with the saps, for it will emit heat and dryness before it reaches the depth of the wound. Small or large amounts should be used, according to the heat of the body and its complexion. In place of euforbius, milk of titimale, laureole or anabula can be used, from which an admirable scammony[47] can be prepared. The weaker substances are resin of pine, apponocus, baura, sea foam, sulfur heated with olive oil, and all medicines which attract the humors to the exterior, such as ferments, etc. I see merit in these, because they attract well by attracting from the depths. Turpentine, moreover, is among the best substances and the one with which we commence treatment.

There are eight kinds of glutinous substances[48] that can be applied in nerve wounds: Resin of pine, resin of fir, resin of poplar, resins derived from the areca tree, the resin known as Colfonia, white pitch known as turpentine derived from the white pine, Mellisa resins, olive resin, and those said to originate like sap from sap-giving trees. All these eight kinds can loosely be termed glue, and we often purify them when we wish to diminish their sharpness.[49] In those nerve puncture injuries where the wound openings have closed off, medicaments must be hotter, drier and more bland than those applied to a nerve incision, so that they may more quickly penetrate to the depths. But when putrefaction occurs in these [62^{v}] wounds, the praiseworthy drugs are dogstone and broomrape meal.

Item. Experienced physicians agree that a sap with calamine and oil comforts in severe pain.

According to Galen, care must be taken that medicines be bland, tepid, dry and without painful properties. To start with, when the wound is uncomplicated we use the white glue, i.e., gum of fir in which is dissolved powdered earthworms dried in the shade. Over this, heat is placed. If, however, the wound is consoli-

[46]caro
[47]scamonea
[48]species glutini
[49]aceritas

de oppoponaco, et de piretro et castoreo, et aperiatur locus;et purgatione cauterizetur universali precedente.)

Medicamen magistrale et galieni quod valet (Galieni quod mirabiliter valet) in punctura *ad removendum* (nervorum in removendo) dolores. Rx: *serapini* (rasine pini), terventine, euforbii, cere ana dr. i;olei rosati dr. ii. Fiat unguentum.

Item oleum balsamin[um]*i*. *Propter* velocitate*m* sue resolutionis cum sit subtile valde et non cum multa calefactione facit idem.

Unguentum *pro punctura nervi magistrale per nos expertum* (per me expertum ad puncturam nervi). Rx: *euforbii bene pulverizati unc. i; resine pini unc. iii; terbentine lote bene et exsiccate vel de colate ab aqua ad ignem vel ad solem picus navalis unc. ii; serapini unc.iii; cere et olei quantum sufficit. Fiat unguentum.*

(Aliud medicamen Rx: olei rosati unc. iii acatie pulverizate M. i. Inungatur locus circumsirca). Rx: euforbii bene pulverizati unc. i; resine pine unc. iii; terventine lote bene cum vino albo vel aqua et decolati ab aqua ad ignem vel ad solem piscus navalis unc. ii; serapini ss unc; et olei quantum sufficit. Fiat unguentum.)

Emplastrum quod convenit in punctura (nervorum ponendo ipsum) supra unguentum *magistrale optimum* (mirabile). Rx: farine fabarum, ordei fenugreci *ana* M. i; pulveris florum; camomille; mellioti, absinthii calamenti sticados arabici ana M. ss; mirr[h]e unc. i; *mellis* (melle) unc. ii; olei *camomille* (camomellini) unc. ii; vini cocti *quod* (quantum) que sufficit ad distemperandum. Fiat emplastrum.

Unguentum divinum *a deo datum* et est *magistrale* (mirabile) *quod* (et) valet in nervis et hoc tam disco[o]pertis quam in punctura, *et non discopertus* et est satis liquidum in forma et habe[t] ipsum (pro secreto) *quia est de nostris secretis. Rx: olei vicii sive lacrimum* (id est lachrymi) unc. i; olei rosati unc. ss; mellis rosati unc. ii. Aliqualiter decoquantur ad ignem lentum et postea reserva. *In aliqua vase ligneo bene in cerato ut non possit penetrare pissidem propter suam subtilitatem.*

Unguentum *aliud magistrale quod dicitur unguentum* de sandara*ch*a, *quod* (et hoc quia) mirabiliter valet in nervis. Rx: cere albe unc. iiii; terbentine lote unc. ix; masticis unc. i; vernicis, sarcoco*l*de, thuris ana dr. vi et fiat unguentum *mala satum* (malaxatum) in forti aceto vel in bono vino montano albo, et *habe ipsum per secreto tam bonas operationes facit* (est optimum et mirabile) in omnibus *vulneribus carnificatiotivum* (foraminibus carnis) et nervorum.

Unguentum quod convenit in punctura nervorum (mirabile).

dated,[50] then dessicatory substances are indicated in accordance with the complexion and amount of pus. A moderate heat-generating substance is this. Rx: flowers of camomile, wormwood, pennyroyal of each 1 fistful; beanmeal, lupine meal of each 1 ounce. Make a poultice. Boil the ingredients in lye and, if you follow directions, pain will completely cease and you will be honored.

(If, in truth, facial spasm is present, anoint the occiput with oil brought almost to the boiling point, oil of euphorbium, oil of opponacus, oil of pellitory of Spain, oil of castors. Expose the area and cauterize by purging in the usual way.)

A Galenic medicament of wonderful value for removing the pain in nerve punctures. Rx: Resin of pine, turpentine, euphorbium wax of each 1 dram; oil of roses 2 drams. Make an ointment.

Item. Balsam oil with its swiftness of healing powers does the same, since it is very bland and not excessively hot.

An ointment I consider excellent for nerve punctures. Rx: well-ground euphorbium 1 ounce; resin of pine 3 ounces; well-purified and dried turpentine or naval pitch heated by boiling water or the sun 2 ounces; serapin one half ounce; wax and oil of sufficient quantity. Make an ointment. (Another ointment. Rx: Oil of roses 2 ounces; powdered acacia 1 fistful. Anoint the area.)

A wondrously effective poultice for nerve punctures, to be placed above the ointment. Rx: bean meal, fenugreek meal 1 fistful; powdered flowers of camomile, meliot, wormwood, lavender, calamine of each half a fistful; myrrh 1 ounce; honey 2 ounces; oil of camomile 2 ounces; boiled wine of sufficient quantity to dissolve. Make a poultice.

A wonderful, divine and effective ointment useful for nerve injuries, be the nerve cut or punctured. It has a liquid consistency and is secret. Rx: Vetch oil, i.e., sap 1 ounce; oil of roses half an ounce; red honey 2 ounces. Cook over a slow fire and store it for future use in a sealed wooden container, so that the strength cannot escape.

Scandaraca ointment is of singular value for nerve injuries. Rx: white wax 4 ounces; purified turpentine 9 ounces; mastix 1 ounce; vernix, sarcocella, frankincense of each 6 drams. Make an ointment, softening it with a strong vinegar or good white moun-

[50] compositum

Rx: olei communis dr. iii; croci scrup. i; et calefac ad ignem oleum cum croco, *et prohice* (proiice) in punctura et superpone de coto madefacto in oleo *et oppone puncture.* Item supra dictum cotum pone unum tale unguentum. Rx: unum vitellum ovi mixtum cum oleo calido et croco, et cum stupa supra locum actu calidum vulneri appone. Quia istud est mirabile mitigativum doloris in vulneribus nervorum.

Unguentum ad incisionem nervorum. Rx: vermes terrestres per optime *pista* (pistatos), et supra labia vulneris per tres dies pone, quoniam quid mirabile videbis in operatione sua.

Mirabile remedium ad removendum magnum dolorem nervorum, sive fuerit punctura sive incisio vel quomodocumque loco. Rx: unum *bistum* (viscum) fili crudum decoctum in cineribus, et sic calidum pone supra locum.

Unguentum *ad mitigandum dolorem* (mitigantium doloris) in puncturis *nervorum.* Rx: care, olei, communis salis ana unc. i; terbentine unc. ii; *liquifiat* (liquifacit) et (omnia) incorporentur optime *in*simul omnia in formam unguenti de quo calido super locum dolentem ponatur et mitigabitur.

Unguentum aliud ad removendum dolorem ubicumque locorum fuerit. Rx: panem albissimum calidum cum egreditur *ex* (de) furno, sume medu*l*lam, et sic calidam pone in lacte, et quando erit bene mollificata exprime et loco patienti appone et videbis mirabilia.

Unguentum ad confortandum nervos incisos post vulneris consolidationem *et est mirabile.* Rx: serapini, castorei ana unc. i; ireos unc. i; euforbii unc. ii; olei anetini, et de cucurbita omnia simul incorporentur cum predicto oleo et *suficienti* cera. Fiat unguentum [63r]

Emplastrum conveniens in qualibet incisione nervorum super unguentum. Rx: farine farbarum, farine ordei, farine fenugreci ana M. i; fermenti exiccati ad formam pulveris unc. ii; florum cammomile, et calamenti, et sticados arabici, et assari, et absinthii ana M. ss; olei olivarum novi, si fuerit hyems, si fuerit estas olei rosati lib. ss; vini *cocti* quantum sufficit. Fiat emplastrum *nam istud emplastrum est mirabile* (et est admirabile in removendo dolorem).

Emplastrum (aliud) mundificatium (et) abstersivum in vulneribus et ulceribus nervorum. Rx: terventine bene ablute cum vino albo et adde de melle apum ana unc. i; vitella ovorum duo et bene misce insimul et adde farine ordei et farine fabarum quod sufficit ad incorporandum.

tain wine. This is excellent and wonderful for all flesh or nerve perforations.

A wonderful ointment for nerve punctures. Rx: common oil 3 drams; saffron 1 tablespoon. Heat the oil and saffron over a fire and pour into the puncture. Over this, place cotton moistened in oil. Item. Over the cotton, apply an ointment such as this. Rx: one egg yolk mixed with hot oil and saffron. Place with a hot stupe above the wound. This is wonderful for easing nerve and wound pain.

An ointment for nerve incisions. Rx: Well-ground earth worms. Place above the wound edges for three days, and you will see an excellent result.

A wondrous remedy for removing severe nerve pain when a puncture or some sort of incision is present. Rx: one viscid drop-wart cooked in charcoal. Place hot above the wound.

An ointment for relieving pain in puncture injuries. Rx: wax, oil, salt of each 1 ounce; turpentine 2 ounces. Liquefy and incorporate all ingredients simultaneously to form an ointment. Place hot above the wound. You will see wonderful things.

Another ointment for removing pain whenever it may exist. Rx: Hot white bread straight from the oven. Remove the crust and put the rest of the hot bread in milk. When it is well softened, apply over the patient's lesions for an excellent result.

An ointment for comforting incised nerves after the wound has healed. Rx: serapinum, castor of each 1 ounce; iris 1 ounce; euphorbium 2 ounces; oil of dill and oil of gourd. Mix all with the right amount of oil and sufficient wax. Make an ointment. [63^r]

A poultice appropriate for any kind of cut nerve, to be placed above an ointment. Rx: bean meal, barley meal, and fenugreek meal 1 fistful; leven dried out to a powdery consistency 2 ounces; flowers of camomile, calaminth, lavender, asarabacca and wormwood of each half a fistful; olive oil—fresh olive oil if it be winter and oil of roses if it be summer—half a pound; wine of sufficient quantity. Make a poultice. Excellent for removing pain.

Another poultice for cleansing and debriding wounds and nerve ulcers. Rx: Turpentine, diluted well with white wine and bees honey of each 1 ounce; yolk of two eggs. Mix well, adding barley meal and bean meal enough for incorporating.

An ointment for paralytics and gout sufferers. Rx: Leg marrow or the fat of an ass, cat fat and vulture fat. Add a little white wax. Make an ointment and anoint the lesion frequently. It is of

Unguentum in paraleticis et arteticis, sive podagricis mirabile. Rx: medul[l]e (crurium), asini *medulle stae* (vel)*sive* (pinguedinis ipsius) pinguedinis ga*tt*i et *asungia* (pinguedinis) vulturis addita *modico* (pauca) cera alba (et) fiat unguentum de quo sepe locus ungatur et valent h*o*(e)c maxime contra indignationem nervorum et *in attritione* (eorum attritionem) et punctura[m] et inflammatione[m] *propter* (et) percussionem nervorum.

Emplastrum mundicativum abstersivit in vulneribus et ulceribus nervorum. Rx: terbentine bene ablute cum vino albo et adde de melle apum unc. i; vitello ovorum duo et bene misce insimul et adde farine ordei et farine fabarum quod sufficit ad incorporandum.

Unguentum (aliud) in paraleticis et arteticis et generaliter in qualibet passione nervorum ibi non *cadat* (cadit) maxima solutio continuitatis et valet *super* (supra) omne unguentum *unde primo* (in principio). Rx: origani calamenti, rute, salvie, primule veris, calendule, *sanamunde* (canamunte), savine ana M. i; piperis, euforbii, piretri ana M. ss; omnia pulverizata conficiantur postea cum unguento arogon *permiste et loco* (et locum) *patienti* (patientem) unge. Deinde quod est melius. Rx: vulpem *excorticatam* (excoriatam) et ab intestinis mundatam et ex rebus supradictis ventrem *impletur et bene* (imiple et) suatur et suaviter ad ignem volvatur, *quod distillantis accipiatur*, et postea cera rubea admisceatur *et usui reservetur* (in eo quod ab ea distilaverit).

Aliud *nobile* (singularissimum) medicamen facta[m] universali evacuatione per flobo*th*omiam *quod* (et) valet in debilitatione nervorum post consolidationem in *paraliticis* (paraleticis). Rx: lacertam (seu stelionem) *viride* (viridem) excortica[t] ipsam et frige in oleo communi vel rutaceo, et sic calida[m] appone supra locum. Sed aliqui accipiunt catulum parvum, et ranas aquaticas et lumbricos terrestres et *lacertam* (stellionem). Et scindunt catulum per medium *abiectis* (deiectis) intestinis et misce omni *in*simul et appone aliquantulum de oppoponaco et imple catulum his rebus *et claude ipsum* et sue ipsum, et assa ipsum *ut* (tanquam) esset agnus et calidum supperpone loco, et est mirabilis medicina.

Unguentum de vulpe ad nervos contractos. Rx: olei serapini, olei iuniperi, olei de terbentina ana unc. vi; adipis ursi, gati *tapsi* (tassi), mellis crudi, cere rubee ana unc. ii; armoniaci, asse fetide, galbani, serapini, olei petrolei ana unc. i; *asungie* (axungie) porci unc. ii; piretri, gentiane, piperis longi, *bacelauri* (bacarum lauri), aristologie, castorei, *mirre salis* (mirasolis) ana dr. ii; euforbii,

great value in nerve indignations, attrition, puncture, swelling and percussion.

Another ointment for paralytics, gout-sufferers and, in general, for any nerve disorder where complete transection has not occurred. When used early, it is superior to the other ointments. Rx: Pennyroyal, calaminth, rutin, sage, primrose, marigold, cinnamon, savin of each 1 fistful; pepper, euphorbium, pellitory of Spain of each half a fistful. Pound all together to a good consistency, adding aragon ointment. Anoint the lesion of the patient. Thereafter, this is even better. Rx: A skinned and eviscerated fox. Stuff the foregoing ingredients into the abdominal cavity and suture it. Then gently barbecue. Afterwards, mix red wax with the drippings.

Another extraordinary medicament for use following a phlebotomy evacuation. It is useful for debilitated nerves in paralytic patients following wound consolidation. Rx: Ordinary or spiny lizard. Skin it alive and roast it in common oil or root extract. When hot, place it above the lesion. Others use a small puppy dog, frogs, earth worms and lizards. The dog is cut in the midline and eviscerated. Mix the foregoing ingredients, adding a little oppononacus. Then they fill the belly of the pup with these ingredients, stitch the belly and roast the pup in the manner that one roasts a lamb. Place it hot above the lesion. It is a wonderful remedy.

A fox salve for pinched nerves. Rx: Serapinum oil, oil of juniper, oil of turpentine of each 6 ounces; fat of bear, cat, badger, crude honey, red wax of each 2 ounces; armoniac hot and acrid, galbanum, sebapanum, mountain oil of each 1 ounce; pork fat 2 ounces; pellitory of Spain, gentian, long peppers, bayberries, castor and sunflower of each 2 drams; euphorbium, nigelle, mustard, laudanum, mastix of each 1 ounce. Clean the above, place in a fox and roast it over a fire. Cook until the fox is well consumed with all the above-mentioned.

Another useful ointment for nerve compression. Rx: Fat from the badger, vulture, toad, snake, an old cow's leg and porcine jaw marrow of each 3 ounces; frog fat, moist wool, mucilaginous fenugreek, flax seed, wild mallows of each 3 ounces; bdellium, armoniac, galbanum, opoponax, euphorbium and castor of each half an ounce; oil of camomile, oil of costus, castor oil, oil of nardine spice, oil of laurel of each 1 ounce. Make a mucilage with the syrup of elder root half a pound; fresh wax 2 ounces; fat of hare

nieglle, sinapi[s], laudani, masticis ana unc. i; omnia *ergo* summo modo terantur et ponantur in vulpe ad ignem, et coquantur donec vulpis bene consumpta sit cum omnibus supradictis rebus.

Aluid unguentum *ad* (in) contractione*m* nervorum (per me) expertum. Rx: adipis tassi vulturis, *rana bufi* (terabufii), adipis serpentum, adipis cruris vaccini antiqui, medulle mandibule porci (ana iii); *adeps* (apidis) anatis *ysopus humida* (ysopi humide) ana unc. i;mucillaginis fenugreci et simins lini et maluavisci ana unc. iii; bdel[l]ii; armoniaci, galbani, oppoponaci, euforbii, castorei ana unc. ss; olei *camomile* (camomellini), olei costini, olei castorei, olei nardini, olei euforbii, olei laurini ana unc. i; et fiat mucillago cum suc[c]o radicis ebuli libra ss; cere nove unc. ii; adipis vulperis;adipis leporis ana unc. i;olei de terbentina; olei vulpini ana unc. i; adipis asini et medule cruris eius adipis anseris, unguenti martiatonis, et aragonis, agrippe, dialtee, butyri ana unc. i; et fiat unguentum pro divitibus.

Allud *unguentum et* medicamen nobile ad contractum nervum, seu ad extendendum nervum *quod est valde* expertum. Rx: de maluavisco quantitatem, quam vis, et ablue ipsum in *lisivio* (lixivio) postea depone [63ᵛ]a lisivio (luxivio), et *dimicte* (dimitte) sic stare per noctem deinde cum illo lixivio coque et cum erit bene coctum *removeas* (remove) illam pelliculam subtilem superiorem postea ter[r]e, deinde adde pulverem santoline, et simul bene incorpora, et super locus ap[p]one et vide bis bonam operationem.

Aluid unguentum ad debilitatem nervorum a quacumque causa sit preter *ex* (ab) incisione. Rx: dialtee, mucilliginis, fenugreci, et seminis, lini, enule ana unc. ss; unguenti agrippe, unguenti marcia*n*tonis, terbentine, lote, pinguedinis anatis, tassi, ursi ana unc. v;olei vulpini, olei laurini, oleo de yreos, Betonice ana dr. ii; cere viridis quantum sufficit, (et) fiat unguentum molle, et unge locum patientis *dolentem et debilitatum.*

Unguentum aliud ad debilitatem nervorum magistrale et secundum Almansorem in novo. Rx: castorei dr. ii; olei de *narcisco*, (narcisco); olei de lilio ana unc. ii; mirr[h]e, oppoponaci ana dr. ss; euforbii dr. iii; cere albe quod sufficit. Fiat unguentum molle.

Aliud unguentum ad idem ad unguendum *supra* spinam *ad spasmum* (in spasmo). Rx: olei casterei ana unc. i; cere quod sufficit. Fiat unguentum cui addatur unguentum de gummis ad pondus omnium.

Unguentum conferens membro debilitato per incisionem nervorem. Rx: savine unc. ss; dactili maturi unc. i; enule compane unc.

and fox of each 1 ounce; oil of turpentine, wolf oil of each 1 ounce; fat of an ass, marrow of the leg of a fat goose, marciaton ointment, aragon, agrippe, dialtee ointment, butter of each 1 ounce. Make an ointment. Suitable for the wealthy patient.

Another wonderful and well-tested medicine for nerve contrition or nerve stretching. Rx: Wild mallow, as much as desired, and clean with lye. After, [63v] remove it from the lye and allow to stand overnight. Then boil in the lye until hot, removing the soft scum at the surface. After, stir and add powdered wormwood, incorporating well. Apply over the lesion for a good effect.

Another salve for debilitated nerves resulting from all causes except laceration. Rx: Marshmallow, mucilaginous fenugreek, purified turpentine, frog fat, badger fat, bear fat of each 5 ounces; oil of fox, oil of laurel, oil of iris, betony of each 2 drams; green wax of sufficient quantity. Make a soft salve and anoint the lesion.

Another ointment for debilitated nerves, according to Almansor in the ninth section. Rx: Castor 2 drams; oil of narcissus, oil of lilies of each 2 ounces; myrrh, oponanax of each half an ounce; euphorbium 3 drams; white wax of sufficient quantity. Make a mild ointment.

Another medicament for comforting nerves and removing pain. Rx: The herb called hemlock and dwarf elder. Boil over hot charcoal and apply these herbs often to the limb, insuring that they are very hot.

A verified experiment for removing pain for incised nerves, wherever their location. Rx: Sulfur, wine boiled with old common oil. Place hot above the nerve to assuage pain.

Item. For removing the pain of puncture wounds and for dilating these punctures. Rx: Boiling euphorbium oil or, if not available, use hot common oil. Place in the puncture.

Item. Take flaxseed meal, honey, yolk of egg. Place over the lesion.

Item. Note that for removing nerve pain, oil from the egg yolk does this.

Item. Lavender oil is useful for nerve pain of the joints. Insure that it is hot to comfort the nerve.

For joint pain, especially pain in in the knee joint, this is a wonderful remedy. Rx: Bull dung mixed with vinegar. Apply over the lesion.

Item. Charnedrys cooked with honey applied to the skin also cures pain.

iss; mirrhe, [h]ypoquistidos, galbani ana unc. ss; balaustiarum, corticum granatorum ana unc. vi; seminis *rosarum* unc. ss; masticis, *almugat, id est, bdelium* (bdelli) ana unc. i; olei mirtini lib. ss; cere citrine quod sufficit, *gume* (gummi) misceantur cum oleo mirtino et pauco aceto, *et* fiat unguentum in modium ceroti, *appone supra membrum.*

Aluid unguentum, ad idem conferens (in) membro debilitato. Rx: cere citrine dr. i; olei de ben dr. ii; masticis, storacis ana dr. ss; croci scrup. i. Fiat unguentum.

Aluid ad idem. Rx: *martiatonis* (marciantonis), aragonis, agrip[p]e, (olei lauri), olei terbentine ana unc. i; olei castorei; olei de lilio ana unc. ss; cere quod sufficit fiat unguentum.

Unguentum (aliud) ad *contractionem* (contritionem) nervorum et dolorem ipsorum absque incisione. Rx: cere, *butiri* (butyri) ana unc.ii; vitella ovorum vii; colofonie, masticis armoniaci, salvie, ana unc. iii; adipis anseri[s] unc. ii; Fiat unguentum.

Aluid medicamen ad subtiliandum nervos, *incisos* et ad removendum dolorem. Rx: herbam que vocatur cicu*th*a et *ebolus* (ebrilus) et fac bul*l*ire inforti cinerata et tene membrum multum in dictis herbis *decoctis* (coctis) incinerata et fac *quod omnia* (ut) sint bene calide.

Experimenta verissima ad removendum dolorem in incisione nervorum ubicumque fuerit. Rx: sulfur vinum bul*l*itum cum oleo communi antiquo et calidum super nervo positum sedat dolorem.

Item ad removendum dolorem in punctura et ad dilatandum ipsam puncturam. Rx: oleum euforbii actu calidum et pone in punctura *vel* (et) oleum commune calidum, si non *potest haberi* (potes habere) oleum euforbii.

Item ad idem. Recipe de farina seminis, lini mellis et vitella ovorom confice *et* pone supra. Item nota quod in remotione doloris nervorum oleum de vitellis ovorum mirabiliter removet dolorem.

Item oleum de sticados valet (in), doloribus nervorum *quod fuerit* (fuit) in iuncturis, et habet calefacere et comfortare ipsum nervum.

Contra dolorem iuncturarum et genu mirabile. Recipe stercus bovinum cum aceto mistum loco superpositum valet.

Item camedreos *cocta* (contrita) cum melle et *supra locus apposita* (supposita) curat dolorem anche. Item calamentum decoctum cum vino curate dolorem musculorum.

Emplastro in membro iuncturoso ubi sit dolor causatus a materia frigida. Rx: *florum* (floris) rosarum, camomille, absinthii,

Item. Calaminth boiled with wine also cures pain.

A plaster for the joints when pain is caused by cold substances. Rx: Flowers of roses, camomile, wormwood and calaminth, cooked well in dark wine to which is added 1 fistful of leaven; [64r] oil of cost, oil of camomile of each 2 ounces; barley meal, melissa meal, milium meal of each 1 fistful; liquid potash of sufficient quantity. Make a plaster.

A salve for paralysis and tremor when a hot ointment to the area is indicated. Rx: Olive oil, the oldest obtainable, 1 pound; earthworms half pound. Boil the earthworms in sufficient oil. Then Rx: Elder sap 3 pounds. Mix the elder sap with the aforementioned oil and boil. This consumes the sap, leaving the power in the oil.

Item. Another proved experiment for paralytics and patients having a nerve or extremity tremor. Rx: Good quality white wine 4 pounds. Boil in a cooking vessel to which you add 1 fistful of sage. Continue to boil until only 1 pound remains. Give this to the patient to drink on an empty stomach in several doses of 2 ounces, adding 2 drams of mountain wine, and half a dram of a good ground castor. As I say, let him drink the wine for six days with the total of 2 drams of castor. Thereafter, anoint the region.

A wonderful and unknown ointment for complete spasm. Rx: Cost oil; pepper oil of each 4 ounces; euphorbium oil, brick oil of each 3 ounces; purified turpentine 6 ounces; white wax of sufficient quantity. Make an ointment. It will have a white appearance.

A wonderful ointment for the cure and prevention of nerve contrition and for conforting the joints. Rx: Horse fat; this in itself is a wonderful thing.

Item. For pain resulting from excessive cold or from paralyzed limbs. Rx: Fat from a red cat. This by itself is a wonderful adjuvant.

An ointment for curing pain in joints, muscles and severed limbs. Rx: Syrup of elder root 5 ounces; pig fat 3 ounces. Place these together in the shaft of a reed, seal it well and boil it in water. In the shaft an ointment will remain, with which the patient can be anointed.

Note, *dear son*, lest befall thee what happened to one good man of Padua who sustained a nerve puncture caused by a sliver of iron lodging in the ring finger of the left hand above the medial joint. A certain physician was called, wise and celebrated in his knowledge of theory and full of opinions, although he lacked practical knowledge. Rational in surgery but foolish in the matter at hand, he bade

calamenti bene *coopertur* (coctorum) in vino nigro cui addatur ferminti *sive meganum* [64[r]] *furfuris* M. i; olei costini, olei camomellini ana unc. ii; farina ordei, et farine milice, et farine milii ana M. i; lixivii quantum sufficit. Fiat emplastrum.

Unguentum *quod paralisi et* (in paralesi in) tremore de quo calido inungendo locum *patientis* est optimum. Rx: olei olibarum, de antiquori, quod *possit reperiri* (haberi possit) lib. i; lombricorum de terra lib. ss; Bul*l*iat indicto oleo quantum sufficit. Deinde Rx: lib. iii suc[c]i eblui et *misteatur* (misceatur) cum ipso oleo *et tamen bulliat insimul quod consumatur totus succus et remaneat virtus in oleo*.

Item aluid experimentum probatum in paralesim, et ad tremorem *nervorum vel* membrorum. Rx: lib. iiii vini albi et de meliori quod *reperiri* (haberi) possit, et ponatur in una *anglestaria* (ingristaria) ad bul*l*iendum in qua ponatur de salvia M. i; et tantum bul*l*iat quod remaneat lib. i de quo vino *datar bibere* (da ad bibendum) patienti pro qualibit vice unc. ii stomacho ie[i]uno addendo in illis duabus dragmis vini (alterius vini montani) dr. ss per qualibit vice castorei perfecti, *pisti* sed bibat in sex *vicibus* (diebus) vinum cum dr. iii castorei prout dixi*t*, postea fiat unctio supra locum.

Unguentum mirabile et secretum ad spasmus absolute. Rx: olei costini, olei de piperibus ana unc. iiii; olei de euforbio, olei de lateribus ana unc. iii; terbentine lote unc. vi, cere albe quantum sufficit, et fiat unguentum *molle quod erit album.*

Unguentum mirable ad removendum *et prohibendum* contritionem nervorum, et *multum valet ad conforandum* (comfortat) iuncturas. Rx: pinguedinis equine et ex se sola est res *valde* mirabilis.

Item ad dolorem *causatum* (tamen) a materia frigida, et ad membrum *paraliticum* (paraleticum). Rx: pinguedinem gat*t*i rubri et talis pinguendo ex se sola est *res experta et* magni iuvamenti.

Unguentum ad removendum dolorem in iuncturis et *in* musculis et *lacertis extrematium* (extremitatibus lacertorum). Rx: suc[c]i radicum ebuli unc. v; *asungie* (axungie) porci unc. iii et ponatur ista insimul mista in can*n*onibus arundinum bene obturatorum, et bul*l*iantur in caldario plena aqua bulienti[s], et in canonibus illis fiat unguentum qua ungere *poteris* (possis) locum patientem.

Nota *filii carissime* (amice) ne tibi *accidat* (accidit) sicut (cuidam) bono viro *paduano* qui habebat puncturam in nervo factam ex *ferro minuto* (fero) subtili in manu sinistra et in digito annulari super mediam iuncturam. *Nam* (Et ivit) quidam *physicus sapiens et famosus in sua doctrina et carens experimento et ratione in cirurgia sed stolidus in*

the patient apply such mollifying medicines as plaster of wheat, flour and water, and oil and saffron. Notwithstanding, the hand putrefied and death set in on the seventh day. Spasm followed the putrefaction brought on by the inappropriate application of bad plasters. *So believe that the expert is to be followed in the art.* (Because of this, the instructions of inexperienced doctors are not accepted nor sought after in such illnesses.)

hac re iuxit approximari (stolidus cyroicus, et approximavit) medicinas mollificativas scilicet emplastrum *de* (factum ex) farina tritici, oleo *et* (cum) aqua et croco, sed tandem putrefactam est manus et mortuus est *in* die septima, ex hoc quia supervenit spasmus propter putrefactionem factam ex indebita approximatione mali emplastri, *quia crede quod quodlibet expertus credendus est in arte* (et propter hoc non sunt accipiendi homines imperiti, aut ceratani ad tales passiones).

IIIa

Sequitur *Capitulum* de apostematibus que accident nervis vulneratus.

Cum addicit apostema in vulneribus nervorum tale vulnus non posset esse absque *magno* dolore (maximo). Sed tale apostema *non erit apparens aut occultum* (aut est apparens, aut non) apparent *et* ad extra, tunc *illud arguitur ad extra apparere,* (tumore apparente arguitur) esse bonum signum, et quod materia non sit intrinsecata in prorsitatibus membri nervosi. Sed si sit dolor continuus et tumor non sit apparens, *significat* (arguitur) materiam esse intrinsecam, et absque dubio spasmum futurum *iudicemus* (iudicabimus). Et si dolor ille perseveret mors erit propinqua. Nam si in huiusmodi vulneribus *accidat* (accidit) flegmon, tunc flobatomiam laudamus constante virtute. Sed si tale fle[g]mon sit valde inflammativum ut tangit Galienus in Liber *caragenis* (catagenis) administrentur per eius curatione locali medicine facte cum aceto et lapidibus mineralibus, et iste medicine reperte sunt in secundo tractatu *cathagenis* 3.1, cuius Rx: calcadis [64^{v}] dr. i et quartam et draganti (vini) *dr. viii* ss (et quartam), scorie plumbi dr. ii et corticum thuris dr. iss et galbani dr. i et cere dr. vii, olei dr. *ix* (si) (et) aceti fortis *lib. ii* et quartem terantur medicine sicce sum aceto decem diebus et solvantur ea que solventur et infrigidentur et misceantur omnie in oleo et moveantur (omnia) motu exquissitissimo donec equetor. *Nichil* (Nihil) *vere nocibilius est nervis infirmis quam* (est magis et minus quantum virtus) illud quod est frigidum. Calidum vero est amicum et utile.

(Emplastrum in apostematibus nervorum. Rx: florum camomille, pulegii, calamenti ana M. i farine fabarum, lupinorum ana unc. iii decoquantur in lixivio deinde malaxentur in oleo sambucino camomillino quantum sufficit. Fiat emplastrum).

Chapter IIIa

The following concerns pus occurring in nerve wounds.

When pus occurs in a nerve wound, the wound is never without great pain. The pus may or may not be evident. If externally evident, then a swelling appears, which is a favorable sign, signifying that the suppurative material is not intrinsic in the pores of the nerve shealth.[51] If pain continues without swelling, this signifies that the pus is intrinsic and, doubtless, spasm will be forthcoming. If pain persists, death will supervene. Should phlegmon appear in these wounds, we recommend the ever-reliable phlebotomy with its faithful virtues. If, on the other hand, the phlegmon is very inflammatory,[52] as Galen states in the Book of *Categories*, then administer for the cure of the region medicines compounded with vinegar and mineral stone, the formula for which is contained in the second tractate [64ᵛ] of the *Categories*, i.e.: Rx: Vitriol 1 dram; dragon wine 8 drams; lead slags 2 drams; bark of the olibanum tree 1 dram; galbanum 1 dram; wax 7 drams; oil 6 drams; strong vinegar 2¼ pounds. Mix the dry medicines with vinegar for ten days dissolving all which can come into solution. Then cool and mix everything in the oil, stirring vigorously until a uniform solution is obtained. Nothing is more harmful to the sick man than cold substances. Warmth, in truth, is a useful friend.

A plaster for nerve pus. Rx: Flowers of camomile, pennyroyal, calamine of each 1 fistful; bean meal, lupine of each 3 ounces. Boil in lye, then soften with elder oil and camomile oil of sufficient quantity. Make a plaster.

Another plaster for nerve pus. Rx: Barley meal, fenugreek of

[51]porositatibus membri nervosi
[52]inflammativum

Emplastrum in apostematibus nervorum. Rx: Farine ordei, *farine* fenugreci ana M. ii; olei liliorum alborum et camomillini ana unc. i; vini cocti ad incorporandum *et* fiat emplastrum.

Emplastrum aliud optimum. Rx: calamenti florum, camomille ana M. ii; furfuris frumenti M. i; sulfuris *pistati* (triti) dr. ii; olei rosati unc. iiii; butyri unc. ii; farine ordei M. i; vini montani, quod sufficit ad incorporandum et fiat emplastrum.

Emplastrum aluid, *valde* conveniens *ex* (in) intentione Avicenni in hoc capitulo. Rx: mel[l]is apum unc. iii; cineris *de lignis dulcibus* (lignorum dulcium optime) cribellati M. ii; farine ordei vel farine orobi M. i; aceti ciatum *unum* et lixivii, quod sufficit ad incorporandum, et fiat emplastrum *et* (quod) *a* ponatur actu calidum.

Emplastrum *aluid* secundum antiquos meos magistros. Rx: malvarum M. iii et coquantur in aqua bene, et pistentur factam expressione ab aqua post decoctionem, (et) admisceatur farine ordei M. iss; *asungie* (axungie) porcine et *butiri* (butyri) ana dr. iii;olei rosati quod sufficit.Fiat emplastrum. (Dolor fixus significat humorem de ambulativum ventositatem gravativum que videatur sibi quod sit pondus magnum multitudinem humoris. Primus significat humores malos. Secundas multos. Tertius utrumque. Alius dolor inflammatus videtur homini qui flamma ignis transeat per spatulas suas, et hoc fit in paratis ad febrem, de sanguine fiat flobatomia, et nisi cito fiat difficule est, quod unumque cuadat.)

IV

Sequitur capitulum De attrictione nervorum *et eorum torsione* (Capitulum IV).

Atritio est solutio continuitatis plurium partium numero accidens in extremitatibus musculorumsive partium *nervosorum* (nervosarum). *Torsio* (Tortio) vero importat non integram seperationem iuncture ita tamen evenit quod ligamenta coniungentia ossa valde compatiuintur. Nam ex sententia Galieni sexto de *interioribus* (inferioribus) *et alii* in tegni. Nervus extenditur ad tria significata scilicet ad nervum ad c[h]ordam et ad *ligamenta* (ligamentum) coniungentia ossa. Et similiter hic intendimus in proposito, quia hec omnia membro habent similitudinem inter se, sed non videntur habere unum et idem officium. Nam cum acciderit in nervo absque *vulnere* et apostemate attritio, *primo* facta *universali* evacuatione curetur hec attritio cum eo quod sedat dolorem. Et similiter si hec coniuncta fuerint cum apostemata, non procedas cum eo quod fortiter resolvit, sicut cum lixivio et *similia* (similibus), *quoniam* magnificabitur egritudo sed embroco locum patientem cum oleo communi calefacto continua embrocatione, donec dolor fuerit sedatus, et si tale oleum habeat virtutem resol-

each 2 fistfuls; oil of white lillies and camomile of each 1 ounce; cooked wine for incorporating. Make a plaster.

Another excellent plaster. Rx: Calaminth, flowers of camomile of each 2 fistfuls; bean leaven 1 fistful; ground sulfur 2 drams; rose oil 4 ounces; butter 2 ounces; barley meal 1 fistful; mountain wine of sufficient quantity for incorporating. Make a plaster.

Another similarly useful plaster, according to Avicenna. Rx: Bee's honey 3 ounces; well-sieved ashes of sweet wood 2 fistfuls; barley meal or orobus meal 1 fistful; vinegar and potash water of sufficient quantity for incorporating. Make a plaster and apply quite hot.

Another plaster, according to my old masters. Rx: Mallows 3 fistfuls. Boil thoroughly in water. Grind after the water has been discarded, mixing barley meal half a fistful; pig fat and butter of each 3 drams; oil of roses of sufficient quantity. Make an ointment.

(A steady pain signifies a migrating, windy, reluctant humor which is apparent because of the weight, size or multiplicity of the humor. The first signifies bad humors; the second, many humors, and the third, dispersed humors. Another burning pain occurs in men who feel a flash of fire passing through their shoulder blades. This occurs in those disposed to fever. A phlebotomy of the blood should be performed. Unless this be done quickly, the pain is difficult to treat, since it eludes everyone.)

Chapter IV

Concerning attrition and torsion of the nerve.

Attrition[53] is the disruption of the continuity of various structures, often occurring in the substance of the muscles or the nerves. Torsion[54] implies incomplete separation of the joint, for it so happens that the ligaments which bind the bones suffer with it. According to Galen in the Sixth Capitulum *De Interioribus* and elsewhere in the *Tegni*, the nerve is regarded from three standpoints, i.e., from the standpoint of the nerve, the sinew and the ligament binding the bones. This concept applies here, for although all these structures have similarities among themselves, they do not have one and the same function. When attrition occurs in a nerve without a wound or pus, this attrition can be cured by a prompt overall evacuation, with something that relieves pain. Similarly, if a joint becomes infected with pus, do not proceed with substances which cause vigorous resolution, such as lye,[55] etc., for these increase the sickness.

[53]attritio
[54]tortio
[55]lixivio

utivam et mollificativam erit optimum, sicut est oleum de aneto et ruta, et de alch*an*na. Maluaviscus *vero* (autem) in formam emplastri cum *pistetur* (pistatur), et *ponatur* (ponitur) super nervos attritos est mirabilis. Cepa vero domestica sub prunis decocta, *atque* (et cepa etiam) liliorum alborum curat attritionem absque vulnere et apostemate. Si (autem) fuerit *attrictio* (attritio) cum apostemate et absque vulnere, *tunc regula talis sit* (talis sit regula). Ut medicus inquantum potest laboret in sedatio[ne] *huius* apostematis *talis est ut* (Et sedatio talis apostematis hoc modo fiet. Si) administrentur desuper vinum coctum cum oleo *camomillino* (camomellino) et pauco aceto, et cum quantitate *conveniente* (convenienti) et tepida valde, et aliquando cum intromissione aliquantule quantitatis ysopi humide sive lane *sudice* (succide) *que non fuerit ablute.* Nam si *hec* (attritio) *attrictio* fuerit in iuncturis adhuc labora in sedatione doloris, et ponatur medicamen fortius *aponindo* (componendo) cum eo quod mativiat resolvit, et adhuc cum stipticitate temperata, ut prohibeat*ur* adventum apostematis scilicet circumcirca *in* unguendo cum (oleo) unfancino. In attritione *vero* (autem) quando coniungitur vulnus, tunc necessaria sunt ea que fortiter *exsiccant* (exiccant) aggregando partes vulneris cum strictura et ligature convenienti. Farine fabarum acetum et mel est medicamen [65[r]] bonum, et si vis que fortius sit in *exsicando* (exiccando) pone de farina orobi, et *radix* (de radice) lilii.

Item caro o[b]stracarum est mirabilis. Olibanum mi*r*ra sandaraca valet in *actritione* (attritione) cum vulnere, et si ibi fuerit dolor intol*l*erabilis valet (mixta cum supradictis immiscendo) *vix si emplastratur locus miscendo.*

In curatione vero torsionis nervorum que est dispositio recipientium magis ligamenta iuncturarum non oportet ut approximetur aqua*m*, neque calida*m*, neque frigida*m* sed approximentur olea stiptica *calefacta* (calefactiva), in quibus est virtus aromaticorum et bonorum odorum. Nota quod multi audiunt legendo et non intelligunt *considerando.*

Emplastrum *magistrale et communiter consuetum* (optimum quod communiter approximatur) in principio a practicantibus *et hoc* in attritione existente absque apostemate et vulnere. Rx: albumina ovorum tria; olei rosati unc. ss; pulveris boli armeni[am] et sanquinis draconis et volatilis modendini ana dr. ii; omnia conquassentur optime, et cum fald*el*lis stupeis prius madefactis in vino stiptico nigro, et expressis ab ipso vino et balneatis *in ipso sopradicto* (de

Rather, frequently rub warm common oil[56] on the region, until the pain diminishes. Oils, such as anise, rutin and alkanna, which have the power to loosen and soften, are excellent. Ground mallows[57] in the form of a plaster placed above the attritic nerve has a wonderful efficacy. Likewise, domestically cultivated onions cooked under coals and the bulb of white lilies[58] cure attrition, when such occurs without a wound or pus. If, however, attrition occurs with pus and without a wound, then the rule is this: let the physician do his utmost to cure the pus. The cure of pus is accomplished in the following manner. Above the affected area apply wine cooked with oil of camomile and a small appropriate quantity of very tepid vinegar. Add to this a pinch of moist hyssop or fresh unwashed wool. If attrition is present in the joints, direct your efforts toward easing the pain. Stronger medicaments are then added which mature and resolve. Along with moderate styptics, rub around the wound, for example, oil of unfranc, in order to prevent pus. In cases of attrition when the wound is united, one must apply these desiccating remedies, approximating the edges of the wound with ligatures and appropriate binding. Bean meal, vinegar and honey make good remedies [65r] and, if a more powerful desiccator is required, apply extract of broom rape and lily roots.

Item. Flesh of Mussel[59] is wonderful, and frankincense and sandara is also of value for attrition when a wound is present. If intolerable pain occurs, a combination of the above is of value.

In nerve torsion, where the joint ligaments have enhanced sensitivity, neither hot nor cold water should be used for the cure. Apply instead hot styptic oil. It is aromatic and has a good odor. Note: There are many who read but do not comprehend.

An excellent plaster which practitioners often apply in the beginning of the illness when attrition exists without pus or a wound. Rx: White of three eggs, oil of roses half an ounce; powdered bole armeniac, dragon blood and flying seeds of each 2 drams. Pound everything well. Take a linen stupe, soak it in styptic black wine and squeeze out the excess. Then heat it and place it above the patient's lesion, fastening it with appropriate bindings.

Item. This having been done, the following wonderful con-

---

[56]oleo communi
[57]maluaviscus
[58]alborum liliorum
[59]caro ostracarum

supradicto) emplastro, et calido actu, et supra locum *patientem* (patientis) ordinate [ap]ponatur dicte faldel*l*e, secundum quod tibi videtur cum convenienti ligatura.

Item *ad idem* hoc facto apponatur in fine emplastrum *magistrale* (mirabile) constrictivum, quod vocatur emplastrum de *lonbardia* (lombardia) extensum supra corium cuius descriptio talis est. Rx: mumie unc. i; draganti, gummi arabici ana unc. ss; *gessi* (gipsi) lib. ii; aristologie longe et rotunde, consolide maioris ana unc. i; lentis orobi, calignis furni ana unc. ii; boli armeni, terre sigillate, mirr[h]e, olibani, balaustiarum gallarum ana unc. ss; corticum granatorum, nucum cypressi rosarum ana dr. ii; lapidis *emathithis* (ematitis) unc. vi; visci quercini unc. iii; glutini piscium dr. ii; sanguinis humani, pulveris pil[l]orum *leporis* ana unc. ss; cere unc. viii, terbentine unc. ii; resine pini unc. vi; picis navalis *lib. iii* et fiat cerotum *quod dicitur cerotum de lombardia.*

Item istud *tale* cerotum *multum* valet in crepatis et in quacumque ruptura.

Emplastrum *aluid* (bonum) in sola attritione. Rx: radicum consolide maioris et radicum maluavisci et radicum herbe ungarice, (que est similis maluavisco, nisi quod habet frondes incisas magis subtiliter, et etiam vocatur falconeria) ana pista omnis insimul absque dedoctione, *et supra locum* sic pistata [ap]pone, et est *mirabile* (bonum) remedium.

Emplastrum in *actritione* (attritione) cum apostemate. Rx: florum utriusque rose *asini scilicit* albe et rubee et foliorum cameleunte et rosarum et absinthii et florum ciclaminis et florum peonie et boraginis et rosis marini et florum camomille et cuscute et florum olivarum ana M. ss: farine milii et *miliie* (milice) ana unc. iii; (olei communis recentis unc. iiii); *amurca* (amurce) olei unc. i; vini cocti quantum sufficit. Fiat emplastrum, quod est mirabile ad removendum dolores in omni membro attrito cum apostemate.

Item valet unguentum *diatratum* (dialteatum) et unguentum aragon et unguentum *martiaton* (marciaton) et unguentum agrippe et hoc secundum sua tempora.

Unguentum ubi erit *atrictio* (attritio) cum vulnere. Rx: mellis apum crudi unc. ii; farine fabarum et orobi et pulveris yreos quantum sufficit ad incorporandum ana et adde *modicum* (paululum) aceti, (et fiat unguentum). Item valet unguentum basilicon, et unguentum citrinum, et unguentum apostolicon, et unguentum fuscum et valet unguentum grecum maiuis et minus.

stricting plaster, called Lombard plaster, is applied to the skin. Its description is as follows. Rx: Mumie 1 ounce; dragon wort, gum araby of each half an ounce; gypsum 2 pounds; aristolochia long, round and rather solid, majory of each 1 ounce; lentil, broom rape, chalk of each 2 ounces; bole armeniac, Jerusalem soil, myrrh, olibanum, pomegranate, oak-apple of each half an ounce; granate bark, cyprus rose nuts of each 2 drams; blood stone 6 ounces; mistletoe 3 ounces; pitch glue 4 drams; human blood, powdered rabbit fur of each half an ounce; wax 8 ounces; turpentine 2 ounces; resin of pine 6 ounces; naval pitch 3 pounds. Make a pomade, called Lombard pomade.

Item. The above cerate is also of great value for crepitation and rupture.

A good plaster solely for attrition. Rx: Equal parts of whole root of the majory, wild mallow root, roots of the Hungarian herb—which is similar to wild mallow except that its leaves can be cut more easily and is called "falconeria." Grind all together without boiling and place over the wound. It is a wonderful remedy.

A plaster for attrition in the presence of pus. Rx: Petals of either the white or red rose, leaves of camomile and rose, wormwood, cyclamen flowers, peony, borage, rosemary, flowers of olive of each half a fistful; milium meal, melissa of each 3 ounces; fresh common oil 4 ounces; horseradish oil 1 ounce; boiled wine of sufficient quantity. Make a plaster. It is excellent for curing pain in all attritic extremities when pus is present.

Item. Althea, aragon, marciaton and agrippe ointments are of value in season.

An ointment when attrition and an external wound are present. Rx: Unprocessed bee's honey 2 ounces; bean meal, orobus meal and powdered iris of sufficient quantity for incorporating as necessary. Add a little vinegar (and make an ointment).

Item. Basilicon ointment, yellow ointment, apostolic ointment and black ointment are of value, as is Greek ointment, more or less.

V

Capitulum (Sequitur de) iudiciis et *de extractione* (extritione) nervorum corruptorum. (Capitulum V)

Nervus corruptionem sumere potest, sicut caro, aut propter causam primitivam vel antecedentem, sed *quomocumque sit* (si) in aliqua parte alicuius rami vel frusti ipsius nervi accidat illud, tunc necessarium est ut extrahatur totum *istud* (illud) quod erit corruptum. Sed antequam extrahatur necesse est ut expectetur, hora qua natura segregat putridum a sano, et non extrahatur cum violentia, sed cum habilitate, [65v] unde dicit Avicenna quod oportet ut extrahatur extractione qua extrahitur vena civilis, unde ibi recurre per completiori doctrina.

Unguentum ad extrahendum nervum corruptum. Rx: *terbentinan* (terbentine) cum melle ana, farine lolii quod sufficit ad incorporandum, et fiat unguentum et extendatur supra petiam *est* (et) cit[o]*e actrictionis* (extrahit).

Item valet unguentum basilicon.

Unguentum aliud optimum in corruptionibus nervorum. Rx: succi apii domestici unc. ii; vitellum ovi unum terbentine dr. iii; farine *frumenti* (fenugreci) quod sufficit ad [in]spissandum, et fiat unguentum.

Unguentum aluid *ad idem* in corruptionibus nervorum. Rx: lardonis decolati unc. ii; pulveris florum urtice, et semina interiora peonie et pistanda postentur ana dr. ii; terbentine quod sufficit. Fiat unguentum.

VI

Sequitur Capitulum De *duritie* (diricie) nervorum *atque de* (et) eorum torsione. (Capitulum VI)

Durities (Duricies) nervorum *atque* (et) eorum torsio ut plurimum accidit a vulneribus, aut casibus, et quando premitur sentitur cum eo stupor qui est morbus *officialibus* (officialis) faciens evenire in sensu tactuali nocumentum, aut destructionem aut diminutionem cum tremore si est debilis aut mollificationem si est confirmatur, quoniam virtus sensibilis non solum prohibetur a penetratione sed et motiva prohibetur, quamvis in quibusdam horis inveniatur stupor absque difficultate motus propter diversitatem nervorum motus et sensus.

Chapter V

The following concerns the indications for drawing[60] a corrupt nerve.

The nerve, like flesh, can become corrupt from either primary or antecedent causes. If corruption occurs in any part, branch or division of the nerve itself, then it is necessary to draw[61] the whole nerve, which will otherwise become corrupt. But before drawing, one must await the hour when nature separates putrefication from the sanies. Then one must draw not vehemently, but with skill. [65ᵛ] Concerning this, Avicenna states that the material is to be removed as "veins of a citizen" are let. Refer to his text for more complete doctrines.

An ointment for drawing corrupt nerves. Rx: Equal parts of turpentine and honey, darnel meal of sufficient quantity for incorporating. Make an ointment and place above the lesion. It will quickly draw.

Item. Basilicon ointment is of value.

Another excellent ointment for corrupt nerves. Rx: Domestic bee's sugar 2 ounces; one yolk of egg, turpentine 3 drams; fenugreek meal of sufficient quantity for thickening. Make an ointment.

Another ointment for corrupt nerves. Rx: Cooked lard 2 ounces; powdered nettle flowers, inner seed of peony, grind as necessary 2 drams; turpentine of sufficient quantity. Make an ointment.

Chapter VI

Concerning induration and torsion of the nerve.

Induration[62] and torsion of the nerve frequently occur from wounds or accidents.[63] When these conditions progress, they are accompanied by anesthesia,[64] which is illness of the part. Induration causes harm to tactile sensation, destruction, withering[65] and

---

[60]extritio
[61]extraho
[62]duricies
[63]casus
[64]stupor
[65]diminutis

Sed curatio huius egritudinis que est *durities* (duricies) nervorum talis est qualis est curatio apostematum durorum et *porisarcoidi* (pororum sarcoidi) sive arosbodi cum impediunt motum et sensum alicuius membri,propter suam *duritiem* (duriciem) et magnitudinem, oportet attenuari et mollificar secundum duas *revolutiones* (resolutiones) eo modo *quo* (qui) patuit in capitulo de apostemate solirotico, Verum multa ad hec *virulentia reperietur* (valentia reperiuntur) in *au*reolis, secundi canonis Avicenni sicut si in decoctione ciclaminis infundatur spongia, et ponatur super eas *durities* (duricies) et torsiones. Similiter armoniacum cum ex eo *spongia* fit emplastrum cum melle et oleo resolvit *duritiies* (duricies) nervorum et iuncturarum et maxime quando permisce*n*tur cum aceto, et sale baurachino et oleo *et* (de) *alcantice* (alchana) et rosis. Similiter anacardus comfert frigori nervorum, et eius mollificationi et torture et *paralisi* (paralesi). Similiter agnus castus, si ex eo fiat emplastrum, cum foliis suis tortioni *nervorum* comfert. Similiter acorus comfert spasmo stupori et *a trictioni* (contritioni) lacertorum, et si de sua decoctione fiat embrocatio et bibatur. Similiter maluaviscus bene decoctus et mistus cum adipe anseris comfert *duritiebus* (duriciebus)nervorum et tremori et attritioni medii lacertorum. Similiter psilium si fiat ex eo emplastrum (comfert) torsioni nervorum et ipsorum spasmo, et dolori iuncturarum cum dolor ille proveniat *a* (ex) causa calida cum aceto et oleo roso comfert. Similiter narciscus et oleum eius comfert nervis, sed ex radice eius fiat emplastrum, *apostematibus nervorum* (apostemati) (eorum) et nodositati *ipsorum* (eorum) et doloribus iuncturarum valet.

Emplastrum ad duricies nervorum. Rx: *bdellii* (bdellium), *iudaici* (iudaicum) *dissoluti* (dissolutum) in aqua maluavisci *in calida* et radicum altee preparate ana unc. i et bene preparate et pistate et misce insimul. Fiat emplastrum *et emplastetur locus.*

Emplastrum ad *durities* (duricies) et torsiones nervorum. Rx: ceroti de secibus, ceroti de melliloto ana quantum sufficit.

Emplastrum *ad durities et torsionem nervorum* (aliud ad idem). Rx: radices liliorum alborum bona *decoctarum* (decoctas) *in* (cum) vino cocto et *peroptime pistatorum* (bene pistatas) cui addatur *modicum* (paululum) farine fenugreci et fiat emplastrum.

Cerotum optimum in *doloribus neruorum et torsionibus* (duriciebus et torsionibus nervorum). Rx: armoniaci et galbani et euforbii ana unc. i; et aggregentur optime cum fece olei liliorum alborum, et cum *modica* (modico) cere. Fiat cerotum *gummi* sed prius *mollificati* (mollificentur) in oleo liliorum alborum. [66r]

tremor, if the part be weak; or softening, if the part is strong. Not only is the power of sensation prevented from penetrating, but motor function is also impaired, although on occasion anesthesia may appear without impairment of motor function, since motor and sensory function are separate in the nerves.

The cure of induration of the nerve is the same as the cure of pus occurring on the dura or in the pores of granulation tissue[66] or osseous tissue.[67] Torsion and induration impede motor and sensory functions in a structure, in proportion to their induration and magnitude. One must soothe and mollify, according to the two instructions contained in the Capitulum *Concerning Hard Pus.* Truly much of value is found in the contents of the Second Canon of Avicenna, such as the instruction to soak a sponge in boiling cyclamus and place it over the induration and torsion. Similarly, a sponge soaked in armoniac and made into a plaster with honey and oil also resolves induration of the nerve and joints. Its efficacy can be enhanced by the addition of vinegar, salt of baurachus, oil, henna and rose. Similarly, anacar comforts nerve freezing, softening, torsion and paralysis. Pure agnus leaves made into a plaster comforts torsion while gladiolia root boiled down to liniment[68] or given as a drink comforts spasm, anesthesia and pain resulting from the laceration. Similarly, well-cooked mallows mixed with goose fat soothes nerve induration, tremor and attrition in the depths of the limb. Psilium, too, in plaster form, soothes torsion and spasm of the nerves and joint pain. When pain appears from a warm cause, the application of heat with vinegar and red oil comforts. Similarly, narcissus and oil comfort the nerve. From the narcissus root a plaster can be made which is of value for nerve suppuration, nodulation[69] and joint pain.

A plaster for indurated nerves. Rx: Bdellium of Judea dissolved in *warm* water, wild mallow, prepared marshmallow roots of each 1 ounce. Prepare well, grind, and mix. Make a plaster *and place on the affected part.*

A plaster for induration and torsion of the nerve. Rx: Cut-up wax, wax of meliot of each sufficient quantity.

Another similar plaster. Rx: White lily roots. Boil them down

[66]sarcoid
[67]arosbod
[68]embrocatis
[69]nodositas

(Aliud. Rx: oxicroci, ceroti de sordice vasorum apum ana unc. i).

Emplastrum aluid valde conveniens. Rx: seminis prasii *receatis* et per optime *pistentur qua pistata* (pistetur quo pistato) cum vino optimo incorporetur ad ignem, et fiat emplastrum.

Item valet diaquilon cum grummis mollificatum cum oleo liliorum alborum si *erit* (fuerit) durum.

Item valet unguentum sive cerotum de armoniaco descriptu[m] supra in capitulo de scrophulis.

in wine and grind well, adding a little fenugreek meal. Make a plaster.

A good pomade for induration and torsion of the nerve. Rx: armoniac, galbanum, euphorbium of each 1 ounce. Mix these well with the dregs of white lily oil and with a little wax. Make a pomade, softening first with white lily oil. [66^r]

Another Rx: Oxicrocus, discolored pomade standing in a flat-bottomed container of each 1 ounce.

Another poultice of value. Rx: Leek seed, ground up as required, incorporating over fire with good wine. Make a plaster.

Item. Diaqualon is of value. If it is hard, soften it up with gum or white lily oil.

Item. An ointment or pomade of armoniac, described above in the Section *De Scrophulis*, is of value.

II

Commentary on Leonard of Bertapaglia's *On Injuries to Nerves*

Chapter I of the 4th Tractate begins [61^r] with the sentence, "Most precious organ of organs in which sensation is revealed, together with voluntary and involuntary motion. . . .". Variations of this little schema were frequent in classic and medieval medical literature. "Further," wrote Galen,[1] "anatomy clearly shows us that the primary source of all nerves is the brain." Nicolus Physicus[2] in the twelfth century wrote, "The brain, being the most important of the animal members. . .". The second Salerno Anatomy Dissection[3] states, "Among the animal organs, the brain is principal." In Leonard's description, the brain is not only important but "precious," and some suggestion of the author's reverence for the nervous system is reflected in the words "because of the strange, marvelous and occult quality of its majestic nature. . .".

The opening paragraph should be regarded as a tribute to the importance of the central nervous system, rather than a comprehensive review of neuroanatomy. In Leonard's day, the nervous system was known in considerably greater detail than is now commonly supposed. While it is true that the medieval system of anatomy rested solidly on Galenic foundations, one is compelled to acknowledge that Galen's mastery was considerable. In fact, his anatomical exposition is said to fill a volume half the size of Gray's *Anatomy*.[4] In it, Galen identified nearly all the principal gross struc-

[1]Galen, *De Locis Affectis* III.11; VIII.9.

[2]George Washington Corner, *Anatomical Texts of the Earlier Middle Ages*. (Washington, 1927), p. 69.

[3]*Ibid*., p. 55: "Among the animal organs the brain is principal."

[4]George Washington Corner, *Clio Medica: Anatomy*. (New York, 1920), p. 6.

tures of the brain, including the corpora quadragemina, pituitary, fornix, hippocampus,[5,6] and, of course, the vein which bears his name.[7] This was the system followed for twelve centuries and, in truth, the magnificent woodcuts in Vesalius' *Fabrica* (1543) could handily illustrate Galen's text.

The Galenic system, however, must be regarded as a product of the Alexandrian school rather than a unique creation. Through a series of curious circumstances, the wisdom of the Alexandrian tradition survives chiefly in the works of its ultimate disciple who, one remembers, arrived as a newcomer to a city long distinguished for its anatomical excellence.

The introduction to the 4th Tractate, which in the incunabula is called "De Nervis," differentiates the cerebrum from the nucha. *Nucha* is a collective term for the midbrain, medulla oblongata and cervical cord, having been introduced from the Arabic by way of the translations of Constantine the African.[8] The cerebellum was clearly known to medieval surgeons from the work of Galen,[9] but its function was not well understood. The seven pairs of nerves mentioned by Leonard refer, of course, to the cranial nerves. Of the twelve pairs of cranial nerves recognized today, the Galenic system identified only seven.[10] The olfactory and trochlear nerves were mentioned. Gentile da Foligno, Leonard's predecessor, correctly identified the olfactory nerve, but succumbing to veneration for the Galenic seven, rearranged the nerve groupings rather than add to the number. The oculomotor and abducens were regarded as one nerve. Part of the trigeminal nerve was grouped with the facial and auditory nerves, while the glossopharyngeal, vagus, and spinal accessory nerves were held to be one nerve. Today, they are often referred to as the vagus system.

From his experiments with serial transections of the spinal cord, Galen regarded the spinal cord as a second brain.[11] Razi[12] repeats his conclusions. Galen identified 28 pairs of spinal nerves.

---

[5]Adolph Pierre Burggraeve, *Cours Théorique et Practique d'Anatomie.* (Grand, 1840), pp. 32–33.

[6]Friedrich Falk, *Galen's Lehre von Gesunden und Kranken Nervensystem*. (Leipzig, 1871), p. 15.

[7]Galen, *De Anatomicis Administrationibus* IX.1-2; *De Usu Partium* VIII.8-9.

[8]Charles Joseph Singer, *The Evolution of Anatomy*. (London, 1925), p. 79.

[9]Falk, *op. cit.*, for fuller discussion.

[10]Singer, *op. cit.*, p. 56.

[11]Galen, *De Usu Partium* XII.15: Cum enim spinalis medulla velut alterum quoddam cerebrum partibus omnibus quae sunt sub capite.

[12]P. de Konig, *Trois Traites d'Anatomie Arabes*. (Leiden, 1903), p. 9.

Two additional spinal nerves he considered to be terminations of the conus medullaris.[13,14] The entire peripheral nervous system was described by Galen out to, and including, the digital nerves.[15] Leonard alludes to the thoroughness of the Galenic exposition in the expression, "descending to the lower soles of the feet."

From the opening paragraph [61^{r}], so conclusively is the primacy of the nervous system stated that one loses sight of earlier controversy. Aristotle,[16] for example, did not assign supreme importance to the brain but considered it an organ for cooling the heart. Not until the rise of the Alexandrian School was the primacy of the brain recognized.

Returning to the text [61^{r}], we note that the cranial nerves are said to arise from the "coronal commissure." One sees this term in the works of Avicenna,[17] as well as in early medieval writers. "From the commissure of the cranium certain nerves originate which extend to the root of the tongue," writes Niccolus Physicus.[18] Others held that the cranial nerves originated from the ventricles.[19]

Leonard lists [61^{r}] the symptoms resulting from nerve injuries. First, he relates the general symptoms, then specific symptoms. These occur, he tells us in the next breath, with wounds of the sinews as well.

Cold is declared to be a decaying element and cause of putrefaction, because the nerves are created out of humors which can be congealed by cold. The same obtains for moisture. These observations are based on the Aristotelian humoral theory which holds that phlegm, from which the brain and nerves are created, is cold and wet. Heat and dryness, being opposites, are compatible qualities with the nervous system.[20] The danger of congelation by cold was confirmed by Avicenna[21] and seconded by Theodoric[22] and other medieval surgeons.

---

[13] Galen, *De Usu Partium* XII.15.

[14] Walter Creutz, *Die Neurologie des 1–7 Jahrhunderts*. (Leipzig, 1934), pp. 87–89.

[15] Galen, *De Usu Partium* XVI.8.

[16] Singer, *op. cit.*, p. 19.

[17] Avicenna, Canon 1, Fen 1, Doc. 5, Summa 1, Cap. 2.

[18] *Anatomia Magestri Nicolai Physici*, in Corner, *Anatomical Texts of the Earlier Middle Ages*. (Washington, 1927), p. 73.

[19] *Ibid.*: "According to some authorities, all the sensory nerves originate from the cellula phantastica, the motor from the cellula memoralis."

[20] Singer, *op. cit.*, p. 27.

[21] Avicenna, Canon 4, Fen 4, Tract 4, Cap. 1: Et putrefactio quidem festinate ad eos, quoniam ipsi sunt creati ex humiditate quam congelavit frigus.

[22] Theodoric I.15: Solutio continuitatis nervi enim sunt de humidada materia create a frigiditate congelata et conglutinita. Also II.6.

In general, medieval physicians were well aware of the difference between nerve and sinew. Galen[23] discussed the matter in the *De Locis Affectis* and the arguments were repeated by Avicenna.[24] In clinical practice, however, differentiation was difficult. The surgeon's inspection of the wound was limited to the existing laceration, for without local anesthesia, he was unwilling to enlarge the wound to gain exposure. Nor could he rely too heavily on previous dissection for orientation, since dissections were often performed on bodies in varying stages of decomposition. Further, since the dissection had to be completed within four days, as Guy de Chauliac tells us,[25] and, since the courses were few and the attendance large, the dissection was chiefly confined to the larger structures.

But, if the medieval surgeon had difficulty distinguishing tendon and nerve, similar confusion is, at times, encountered even today. It is not unknown for a neurosurgeon to re-explore a nerve injury only to find that a previous surgeon had approximated nerve to tendon!

Leonard [61ʳ], classified nerve wounds in an Arabic format, based on mode of injury. A feeble attempt is made to match type of nerve injury (incision, fissure, etc.) with the nature of the injury. Most of Leonard's terms are unintelligible without recourse to other sources. The Four Masters[26] define an "incision" as the accident which befell a nerve when the wound is transverse. "Fissure" occurs when the wound is longitudinal. When the injury is extensive, the term "concussion" or "contusion" is used. Further, Leonard accepts the Galenic[27] view that paralysis occurs distal to the injury. Similarly, when the nerve is completely transected, flaccidity of the limb results.

An injury to a nerve was regarded by most medieval physicians[28] not only as the cause of distal motor injury, but also of

---

[23]Galen, *De Locis Affectis* III.8.

[24]Avicenna, Canon III, Fen 1, Tract. 1, Cap. 2.

[25]Guy de Chauliac, Tract 1, Doc. 1, Cap. 1, describing Mondinus.

[26]Charles Daremberg, *Glossulae Quatuor Magistrorum super Chirurgiam Rogerii et Rolandi*. (Paris, 1854), Book 1, Cap. 1: Aliquando accidit in nervo, et si secundum latum dicitur incisio, secundum vero longum dicitur fissura; si vero multa et magna, dicitur concussii vel contuso.

[27]Galen, *De Locis Affectis* I.6: Si vero nervi radix afficitur relique partes omnes affecto loco inferiore, nihil afficientur sed solae illae partes resolventur in quas singuli distribuntur.

[28]Avicenna, Canon 4, Fen 4, Tract. 4, Cap. 1: Nervis propter vehementiam sensus corum et continuitatem suam cum cerebro accidunt ex vulneribus dolores vehementes valde, et lesiones valde magnae, sicut spasmus, etc.

retrograde brain damage. To be sure, they held that suppuration and toxicity contributed to the cerebral symptoms, but one perceives an inference that the cerebral complications occur *pari passu* with nerve trauma, i.e., the more severe a nerve injury, the more likely that severe cerebral symptoms would result.

In Leonard [61^{v}], structure is classified according to hardness. The order of hardness, Niccolus Physicus[29] states, occurs with "fat as the softest, flesh is next, then skin, then the sensory nerves, then the motor nerves. . . ligament, then cartilage and finally, bone." This classification is important in guiding the selection of the proper medication, because the harder the affected structure, the stronger the medicine that can be safely prescribed. Note the use of the words *siphac* [61^{v}], peritoneum or dura, and *mirac*, abdominal wall, which entered from the Arabic (Avicenna)[30] in early translations and became established in the anatomy of Modinus.[31]

Before examining the second chapter [61^{v}-64^{r}], one must be aware of the disagreement concerning the treatment of transected nerves (lateral wounds, fissures, scissures, etc.). With regard to punctures (incomplete nerve injuries), there were several aims ("intentions") of treatment. The surgeon must first remove the noxious material; second, promote wound healing; third, keep the wound open; fourth, prescribe proper diet; and fifth, remove noxious humors by such general methods as evacuation, phlebotomies, and enemata.[32] Guy de Chauliac[33] adds to this, "conservation of the part."

Some authorities advocated, others reproved, nerve suture. When the nerve was completely severed, medieval authorities differed on the efficacy of surgery. The Hippocratic School doubted that nerves healed.[34] Galen,[35] for once, is without strong convic-

---

[29]Corner, ref. 18, p. 71.

[30]Avicenna, Lib. 4, Fen 5, Tract. 3, Cap. 1: Multotiens accidit in siphac capitis post curationem cum ferro.

[31]Antoine Portal, *Histoire de l'Anatomie et de la Chirurgie.* (Paris, 1770), vol. 1, p. 211.

[32]Joannes de Vigo, *Practica in Chirurgia.* (Lyon, 1561), Book 3, Tract. 1, Cap. 15.

[33]Guy de Chauliac, Tract. 3, Doc. 1, Cap. 4: Cura igitur vulnerum nervosarum prima, removere extranea, secunda adducere adiniicem labia, tertia in unum conservare, et quarto substantiam partes custodere.

[34]Hippocrates, *Aphorisms* VII.28.

[35]Guy de Chauliac quotes Galen: Ego vidi et audivi in multos nervos et tendones incisos et eos ita restauratos sutura ut postea incredibile videretur; Guy de Chauliac, *Capitulum Universale*, in *Cyrurgia Guidonis de Cauliaco*. (Venice, 1498, *Collectio Cyrurgia Veneta*)

tions. "I have seen and heard about many cut nerves and tendons which have been sutured, and afterward incredible results occurred," he writes on one occasion. Elsewhere, his enthusiasm for nerve suture falters. Guy de Chauliac,[36] in reviewing Galen, concludes, "Notwithstanding that some say Galen does not command to suture nerves, inasmuch that they would not be consolidated and that the poking of the needle is provocative of convulsion. But (save their reverence) Galen has not forbidden it, but if he is silent, yet he has otherwise affirmed it." Further, Guy de Chauliac[37] quotes Avicenna: *Si autem disrupatur in latidudine nervus tunc necessarum est suere ipsum et si non, non conglutinatir*. Lisfranc[38] states, on the other hand, that the treatment of the nerve is the care of the wound itself and advised merely keeping the pores open. In a comprehensive review, Joannes de Vigo[39] in the sixteenth century states that Dinus Florentinus,[40] Petrus de Argellatus, and Hugo de Luca were of the same opinion as Lisfranc. Nerve injuries were not discussed in depth by Theodoric. Concerning Leonard, however, there is little question as to his position. Very clearly, he advised nerve suture, seconding Avicenna. Having thus satisfied the demands of exegesis, we are left to wonder how many nerve sutures were actually performed. I suspect that although indicated, if not recommended, nerve suture was, in fact, rarely undertaken.

Leonard discusses the kinds of medication suitable for nerve wounds. The selection of the cures are based on the Galenic[41] principle of the four elemental qualities (hot, cold, moist, and dry), the secondary qualities (sour, bitter, sharp), and the special qualities (e.g., purgative effect, etc.). Each quality was present in four different degrees. Leonard praises [62^{r}] the use of the saps, citing Dinus as authority. Why he chooses this author is curious. Better than we, he knew that Avicenna[42] had earlier written: *Glutenum albotim est de melioribus medicinis vulnerum nervorum*, commending its

---

[36]Guy de Chauliac, Tract. 3, Doc. 1, Cap. 4.

[37]Guy de Chauliac, Tract. 3, Doc. 1, Cap. 3, *De Incisione Nervorum*.

[38]Lisfranc I.3, *Cyrurgia Parva Lanfranci,* in *Cyrurga Guidonis de Cauliaco.* (Venice, 1498, *Collectio Cyrurgia Veneta*)

[39]Joannes de Vigo, ref. 32, Book 3, Tract. 1, Cap. 15.

[40]Dinus de Garbo of Florence, a student of Arabic medicine and commentator on Hippocrates and Avicenna, died 1327. See J. W. L. Gruender, *Geschichte der Chirurgie*, second ed. (Breslau, 1865), p. 134.

[41]Margaret Sinclar Ogden, *The Liber de Diversis Medicinis.* (London, 1938), p. xviii.

[42]Avicenna, Canon 4, Fen 4, Tract. 4, Cap. 3.

use for children and especially for women. Leonard favors local treatment in the form of ointments and stupes. He extolls the use of lupine products, earlier praised by Arnold of Villanova [43] for nerve afflictions, and by Paulus[44] who recommended their use for head scales. The plasters mentioned in the Four Masters were made of strips of linen.[45,46] The words for drain were *tenta* (Latin)[47] and *stuellis* (Italian),[48] at times used interchangeably. Note the infrequent mention of the iron cautery, the handmaiden of the Arabic physicians. This, despite the fact that Leonard is presenting a commentary on Avicenna!

At the conclusion of Chapter II [64^{r}], Leonard relates a story of a man who sustained a digital nerve injury. He was treated by a "certain physician, wise and celebrated in his knowledge of the practice and rationale in surgery." This was almost certainly a reference to some university colleague and to an incident well known to the academic community. Considering the circumstances, one may be certain that the author's remarks found their way back to the professor in question. Small wonder that Leonard was denied his doctorate until the age of 70! Peter of Tossignano showed more tact in alluding to mishandled treatment. He attributes the malpractice to a barber. (*Et quidam barbitonsor accepit ipsum in cura et tum interfecit.*)[49]

Chapters IV through VI deal with various complications seen in nerve injury when pus forms. The conditions are called attrition, torsion (*torsio*), induration (*duracies*), and constriction. These entities have their origin in Avicenna[50] where, it seems to me, their definition is obscure. Gurlt[51] skims over Leonard's nerve injuries, complaining that the illnesses are incomprehensible to him. It is not unlikely that these terms were not in common use during the four-

---

[43]Edna P. von Storch and T. J. C. von Storch, "Arnold of Villanova on Epilepsy." *Ann. Med. Hist. N.S. 10*:251, 1938.

[44]Ogden, *op. cit.*, p. 84.

[45]Karl Sudhoff, *Studien zur Geschichte der Medizin*, Band 11-12, index.

[46]Walter E. Kunstler, "Asthetic Considerations in Surgical Operations from Antiquity to Recent Times." *Bull. Hist. Med. 12*:27, 1942.

[47]N. Kjaergaard, *Om Drainagen in den aeldre chirurgi.* (Copenhagen, 1892), pp. 84–85.

[48]I. Reichborn-Kjennerud, "The School of Salerno and Surgery in the North during the Saga Age." *Ann. Med. Hist. 9:*321, 1937.

[49]Lynn Thorndike, *Science and Thought in the Fifteenth Century*. (New York and London, 1963), p. 96: "A certain barber undertook the cure and then killed him."

[50]Avicenna, Canon 4, Fen 4, Tract. 2, Cap. 2.

[51]Ernest Julius Gurlt, *Geschichte der Chirurgie*. (Berlin, 1889), vol. 1, p. 860.

teenth and fifteenth centuries. Guy de Chauliac,[52] for example, limits his discussion of nerve injuries to only a few entities. The same is true for Theodoric. Leonard, on the other hand, uses terminology directly from the pages of Avicenna. This is understandable, since his assigned task was to comment on the fourth Fen of the fourth Canon.

Chapter IV [64v-65r] begins with a description of nerve attrition. I have not succeeded in discovering, within the substance of Avicenna, a clear definition of "attrition," but in the marginalia[53] of the incunabula, the editors have providentially defined attrition as a lesion of the nerve associated with pus, but not involving bone. Simply put, this suggests a generalized wound infection in which *inter alia*, the nerve has been injured. The term "torsion" is somewhat more difficult to unravel. The word is used by Avicenna both in his description of soft tissue wounds and bone injuries. Avicenna defines torsion as a situation "when the member is separated from its joints, the separation not complete nor manifest, as when a dislocation is present."[54] I can only surmise that what is meant is a contracture of the limb, which was thought to have resulted from an infected nerve wound. Leonard presents the student a list of valuable medications for these conditions.

Chapter V [65v] deals with "extrication" of a corrupt nerve. Leonard speaks of debriding or incising when nature separates putrefaction from the sanies, or, as one says today, when serosanguinous discharge changes into pus. The author lists a number of ointments, which probably are intended as "drawing" salves. Interestingly, Leonard is remiss in failing to mention constriction (*constrictio*) of the nerve, cited by Avicenna. This occurs when pus, locked up within the nerve wound,[55] cannot find its way to the exterior by spontaneous discharge.

Chapter VI concludes with a discussion of induration (*duracies*) and torsion of the nerve. Leonard appears somewhat unhappy

---

[52]Guy de Chauliac, Tract. 3, Doc. 1, Cap. 3.

[53]Avicenna, Canon 4, Fen 4, Tract. 2, Cap. 2.

[54]Avicenna, Canon 4, Fen 4, Tract. 2, Cap. 1: Contorsio autem est, ut sit membrum separatum a iunctura sica, separatione non completa, neque apparente manefesta (quare est) dislocatio.

[55]Avicenna, Canon 4, Fen 4, Tract. 2, Cap. 2.

both with the terms and his assignment, for he refers the student back to Avicenna. Avicenna states that the cure of induration of the nerve is the cure of hard pus itself.[56] This Leonard repeats almost verbatim. One may therefore surmise that the term, "nerve induration" refers to generalized edema of the tissues when associated with a nerve injury.

[56]Avicenna, Canon 4, Fen 4, Tract. 4, Cap. 7: Et cura duritiei nervorum proxima est curatione apostematum durarum.

III

Leonard of Bertapaglia: Capitulum de Fractura Cranei

I

[68v] *Sequitur Capitulum de fractura cranei. Cum Cupivi veritatem et disciplinam exstimans nullam meliorem rem hominibus in hoc mundo posse percipere. Quia antequam hoc scirem nescivi aut si a deo aut si a fortune hoc accessisset. Verum in arte manuali numquam novi plene peritum ab imperito cum multi doctores atque periti decepti fuerant et maxime in vulneribus nervorum et fracturis capitis quia tot et tanta narrare quanta (a) auctoribus narrata sunt esset quid tediosum audire atque quid confusum et non bene capaxibile pro tunc Fabricio filio meo qui est undicim annorum.*

Ideo in hoc meo opere admodo alium sequar stilum non secutum a meis precessoribus sed allegabo aliquos ubi sunt meo iudicio laude digni et narrabo mirabilia opera nature cum auxilio divino et sequendo modum et regulas antioquorum. Nam in hoc meo opere ammodo intendo facere capitula specialia de unaquaquam egriudine pertinenti cirugico, incipiendo primo a capite declarando de ipsa teorice. Secondo tractando de ipsa practice et optima exempla dando et hoc secundum meam opionem ponendo in formam consilii secundum quod habui in cura et vidi in civitate paduana rome verone venetiis et in alexandria civitate illa in qua Maumeth a saracenis in meca pro deo colitur. Sed iuro per deum vivum et verum crucifixum nullum mendacium fili mi in hoc meo libro tibi facere iuxta meum posse.

Sed primo te oportet haec octo notabilia bene tua mente semper habere si vis esse perfectus cyroicus etiam sic habendo semper preferendus eris aliis.

Primum notabile fac quod tu sis instructus in principiis medicinae et hoc est logica et philosophia si possibile est et per hoc cognosces principia rerum nature. Secundo oportet ut iterum vadas cum experto medico et videas ipsum operari sicut mecum vidisti pluries casus et terribiles sanare et

III

Leonard of Bertapaglia: On Skull Fractures

Chapter I

[68v] The following concerns fractures of the skull.

I have desired truth and knowledge in the belief that man can perceive nothing better in this world. Before coming to this conclusion, I did not know whether this truth would proceed from God or from chance, for frankly in the manual art I could never distinguish the novice from the skilled. Inasmuch as many teachers and experts have been deceived, especially in regard to wounds of the nerves and cranial fractures, were I to recount the numerous and lengthy matters related by our predecessor, this would be tedious to relate, as well as both confusing and incomprehensible to my eleven-year-old son, Fabricius.

In my work I shall therefore follow another method not adopted from my predecessor, citing diverse sources when, in my opinion, they are worthy of praise; and I shall relate wondrous works of nature accomplished with divine aid, following the methods and rules of the ancients. Moreover, in this work of mine, I intend to compose special sections dealing with surgical diseases, beginning with the head. First, I will state the general principles; second, I will present practical considerations, citing what I judge to be the best examples. These I will arrange in the form of counsels, based upon experiences I have derived from treatment and observation in the cities of Padua, Rome, Verona, Venice, Alexandria and in that city known as Mecca, where Mohammed is worshipped as God by the Saracens. I swear, my son, by the living and true God who was crucified, to set down no falsehood in this work of mine, to the best of my ability.

hoc antequam tu operatus fueris. Ratio quia per plura videre tu qui medicum intendis effici devenies in ad surfactionem magisterii et facti medendi.

(Primum arbitror quod oportet eum qui perfectus cyrurgicus esse cupit, multa vidisse. Primum ut habeat logicae ac philosophiae fundamenta, et hoc ut cognoscat naturae principia. Secundo oportet ut vadas cum experto medico, et videas ipsum operari antequam te ad practicandum exponas. Ratio quia videndo terribiles casus, tu vides modum quo utuntur medici in illis sanandis; deinde pervenis ad perfectionem magisterii).

Tertio ut habeas oportet manus leves in operando et expeditas ne facias egrotanti dolorem. *Nam filii mi audivisti illum qui dixit quod habebam manus leves et expeditas quando sibi extrassi illud frustum ossis existens in concavitate cerebri cum illo strumento* [69r]*de carta membrana per parvum foramen ossis fracti et vidisti quod fixi illud strumemtum ad quantitatem unius digiti in concavitate cerebri et de hoc esset testis famossisimus monarca artium et medicine doctor magister Galeacius de Sancta Sophia et magister Nicholaus barbitonsor et magister gerea cerdo et tu fili mi qui omnia haec vidisti. Ratio quia gravitas facit dolorem et dolor est causa attractiones humorum ad locum, quare habe tunc manus leves et expeditas ne inferas dolorem.*

Quatro oportet ut tua [in]strumenta sint bene incidentia, quando oportet aliquid incidere, *et sint sine erugine* et ratio est ex parte duorum, scilicet ne a *malo* (male) acuto [in]strumento, et ab ipsius erugine in membro *in*ponatur dolor, et mala complexio.

Quinto oportet ut sis audax *et non timidus* (intimidus) in operando et incidendo, tamen timendum est incidere ubi sunt venae (sint) nervi c[h]orde et arteriae, et *per hoc ne tibi error acidat fac ut sis sciens clare de anothomia quonim super omnia* (propter hoc ne erres fac ut optime videris anothomiam que est totius mater huius artis, et) fac ut (in primis) sis ingeniosus in operando in tali magisterio, et noli laborare in carne humana sicut fit in ligno vel corio. Ratio quia *judicium divinum in alio seculo exclamabit debete ex tua operatione*. (Quando ex hoc seculo transiveris magna supplicia tibi apponentur, deinde hi tales capiunt malam famam in vulgo quam debemus studere conservare.)

Secto oportet ut sis pius et misericors pauperibus. Ratio quia pietas et misericordia *faciet te a deo et a vulgo esse plusquam dilectus.* (Multum augmentabit tuam famam et libentius egri committent se tibi.)

To begin with, if you wish to be the perfect surgeon, you must always bear in mind these eight notations, and remembering them you will ever be preferred to others.

(The first task of him who wishes to become a good surgeon should be to use his eyes. First, in order to acquire a knowledge of logic and basic philosophy, that you may comprehend the principles of nature.

Second, you must accompany and observe the qualified physician, seeing him work before you yourself practice, for, by observing terrible accidents, you will discern the methods employed by those who treat them and thus attain the perfection of the masters.)

Third, you must command the most gentle touch in operating and treating lest you cause pain to the patient. *Incidentally, you remember when I extracted that bone fragment located in the concavity of the cerebrum with the parchment instrument* [69r] *through a small hole in the fractured bone. You recall, my son, the patient remarking that I had a light and skillful touch. You recall, too, that I inserted the instrument one finger's breadth into the concavity of the cerebrum. This procedure was witnessed by the most famous monarch of the Art, Master Geleatius de Sancta Sophia, doctor of medicine; Master Nicolaus, the barber; Master Gera Cerdo; and by yourself, my son, who saw everything. Clumsiness produces pain, and pain attracts the humors to the site of trauma, wherefore you must have an adept hand, lest you cause pain.*

Fourth, you must insure that your instruments be sharp and unrusted whenever you cut anywhere. There are two reasons: viz. lest pain and a bad complexion[1] be induced in the diseased structure by dull and rusty instruments.

Fifth, you must be courageous in operating and cutting but timid to cut in the vicinity of nerves, sinews[2] and arteries, and, so as not to commit error, you should study anatomy, which is the mother of this art. You should above all perform your surgery cleverly and never operate on human flesh as if you were working on wood or leather, for otherwise, when you depart this life, great punishments will be reserved for you. Furthermore, bad reports are carried back to the public, which must be avoided.

Sixth, you must be kind and sympathetic to the poor, for piety

[1]complexio

[2]chorda

Septimo oportet ut nunquam aliquid *ab aliquo* ex tuo praemio refutes, si aliquid tibi *detur. Ratio quia infirmus ille te putando ipsum non deserere de te melius confidat* (porrigatur quia infirmus maiorem confidentiam de te habebit).

Octo oportet ut nunquam litiges cum infirmis, neque *esse cupidus in omnibus tuis infirmis* (etiam sis nimis cupidus), nisi ex pacto facto petere denarios. Ratio quia *quoniam cupiditas per totum de te honestatet et sic non posses unquam venire ad laudem optimi medici*. (Avaritia est magis ignobile vicium ceteris viciis, et si hoc habebis nunquam poteris ad laudem boni medici pervenire).

II

Capitulum primum de fracta capitis in formam consilii in quo continentur undicem notibiliam. (Sequitur de fractura cranei Capitulum V)

Cum quis *intendat* (intendit) esse *bonus sive* optimus artifex huius magisterii scilicet *scire bene curare fracturas* (curandi fracturam) cranei. *Sed* quamvis *diversi* (plures) auctores (diverse) *diversimode de ipso* tractaverint; attamen *inter ceteros quos perlegi michi placuit insequi dicta Avicenni* (magistrum nostrum sequamur Avicennam). Et quia dicta eius *sunt bona sed* aliqualiter longa *sed non diminuta nec superflua solum brevitur ut menti melius commendetur aliqua sua dicta quae sunt claves in fractura cranei per undicem notabilia totum magisterium brevitar ponam per quae poteris artum curativum absque dubio comprehendere.* (Fiunt ideo brevibus illa attingam; et per XII notabilia totam materiam cranei curandi recolligam, per quae absque dubio poteris fracturam cranei curare. Nota utilia notabilis menti mandanda.)

Primum notabile *sit* (est) istud quod in fractura cranei quantum potes debes prohibere apostemata, ne accidat in cerebro et in panniculis, quia nihil est *ita sevum et* magis prohibens curam fracture et vulneris, et aliarum egritudinum, sicut apostemata. Et ideo ut, possis hoc *iuvenis medicus* (melius) prohibere nota causam apostematis ut eas removere possis.

Prima ergo causa est frigiditas aeris, et aliarum rerum frigidarum approximatarum quae actu sunt frigidae *vel frigiditatis inductivae.* Et idea unguenta et emplastra *et* pulveres et similia debent approximari actu calida, et *iusta* (iuxta) hoc *dictum* (ut dictum

and humility greatly augment your reputation and the sick will more freely commit themselves to your care.

Seventh, you must never refuse anything brought you as a fee, for the sick will respect you more.

Eighth, you must never argue about fees with the sick, nor, indeed, demand anything unless it be previously agreed upon, for avarice is the most ignoble of vices and should you be so inflicted, you will never achieve the reputation of a good doctor.

Chapter II

The first section concerns fractures of the skull, presented in the form of advice. In it are contained eleven points to note. (Here follows Chapter V concerning skull fractures.)

This is written for all who desire proficiency or excellence in the art of curing fractured skulls. Although various authors treat this subject in diverse manners, the author which appeals to me, among others, is Avicenna. Since his excellent treatment is sometimes lengthy, albeit neither impaired nor superfluous, I have merely abbreviated his words in order better to commend to memory those teachings of his which are the key to fractures of the skull. I have condensed the entire mastery of the art into eleven notations, wherefrom, without doubt, you will be able to understand the art of curing. (Commit these useful remarks to memory.)

The first remark is this. In fractures of the skull do as much as possible to prevent pus from occurring in the brain and membranes. Nothing is worse than pus in the cure of fractures, wounds and other diseases. Similarly, that the young physician may more easily prevent and remove them, note the causes of pus.

The first cause is cold air or anything else extremely cold, *or cold-producing* applied to the head. Therefore, diverse ointments and plasters and powders, etc., should be very hot when applied. In connection with this dictum, Avicenna, best of all, states this: in the management[3] of one and all head wounds, you must greatly fear cold, even in summer, for great is the danger.

---

[3]dispositio

est) in textu *per* optime dixit Avicenna. Et in huiusmodi quidem dispositione scilicet capitis vulnerati *ymo* (immo) in omni dispositione scilicet vulneris capitis, oportet *ut* vehementer caveatur frigus, *etiam* in aestate, quoniam in eo est timor magnus.

Secunda *causa* est res ag[g]ravans vel pungens, ag[g]ravans potest esse os depressum vel licinium id est, tenta vel alia quae approximantur indebite, ut puta, si approximaretur emplastrum nimis ponderosum. Et *ideo* docet Avicenna *volendo* (volens) medicum corrigere, quod si frustum ossis pungens sit quod cito removeatur, *quia nisi cito removeatur dolor continue congenerabitur. Et eodem modo removenda est gravitas aliarum rerum* (et ne ponderosa res approximetur), et propter hoc dicit Avicenna quod ponatur pannus subtilis secundum quantitatem [69v] ossis remoti. (Et propter hoc nota) *adverte* quod moderni utuntur panno de *sirico* (syrico) subtili de grana; quia plus comfortat, ut *dicit* (ponit) Avicenna in libro de viribus cordis (docens) quod syricum confortat cor et talis pannus debet esse amplior foramine ossis ne ingrediatur sub osse.

Tertia cause est malum regimen in sex rebus non naturalibus. Avicenna tamen exemplificat de cibo et potu, et dixit de multitudine cibi. Et propterea Avicenna *maxime* exemplificavit de cibo et potu, quia si immoderate *summatur* (sumitur) multum sunt causa apostematis, quia stante fractura cranei virtus digestiva stomaci, et aliorum membrorum est debilitata, unde nutrimentum non bene convertitur. Et ideo multa superfluitas generatur que est casa apostematis, et eodem modo intelligas de potu. Nam hoc idem *expressit Avicenna* (expressum est ab Avicenna) prima tertii in capitulo de soda et in capitulo de *Karabito* (carabito); quia vinum prohibet curam et est causa apostematis *pro quanto* (quia) ad caput evaporat.

Quarta causa est occulta, secundum Avicennam et res occulta secundum ipsum est *illa* (ista) que a vulgaribus non est *nota nec* (neque) infirmo, licet aliquando perito medico sit manifesta, et hoc potest esse repletio humorum, vel debilitas cerebri, vel debilitas alterius membri *mandantis* (mandatis) et ad insinuandum quod Avicenna per causam occultam intelligat repletionem humorum patet dum dicit fiat flobotomia et removeatur causa illa occulta.

Secundum (Aliud) notabile sit istud quod Avicenna in fractura cranei dicit apostemata calidum curari, et loquitur continue de apostemate calido, *et non de frigido. Nam modus curativus apostematis calidi ponitur prima tertii in capitulo de Karabito. Sed Avicenna facit hoc tractando de apostemate calido*, quia raro potest fieri apostem frigidum

The second cause is an object which compresses[4] or pierces[5] the brain. Heavy things depress or cut the bone, as, for example, a drain[6] or heavy plaster or anything else inappropriately applied. Thus Avicenna, wishing to correct the doctor, teaches that if bone fragments pierce, they should be quickly removed, for pain will otherwise continue. Other heavy things should likewise be removed. One must be careful not to apply a heavy object. Instead, Avicenna teaches, a soothing dressing[7] should be applied in proportion [69ᵛ] to the quantity of bone removed. In connection with this remark, contemporary physicians favor a syrian covering of soothing grain which is most comforting. As Avicenna states in his *De Viribus Cordis*, "syrian" soothes the heart, but such a dressing must be larger than the bone defect, lest it sink beneath the bone.

The third cause is a poor regime in the six unnaturals. Avicenna furnishes examples of food and drink, discusses various foods, and cites examples of food and drink, which, if immoderately consumed, can be the cause of pus. For when a fracture of the skull is sustained, the digestive function of the stomach and other structures are weakened, so that nourishment is not well digested.[8] This results in the generation of a copious discharge,[9] which is a cause of pus. The same applies to drink. The latter is discussed by Avicenna in the first part of the third section *De Soda* and in the section *De Carabito*, wherein he states that wine prevents a cure and is a cause of pus, for it rises up[10] to the head.

The fourth cause is occult. According to Avicenna, an occult thing is that which neither the ordinary man nor the patient can identify, although at times it is evident to an experienced physician; for here there can be a plethora of the humors, weakness of the brain or weakness of other given structures. To show that, from occult causes, Avicenna knows a plethora[11] of humor to be revealed, there is evidence in his statement, "Let there be a phlebotomy to remove the occult cause."

The second remark is this. Avicenna in his *De Fractura Cranei*

---

[4]res aggravans
[5]pungens
[6]tenta
[7]pannis subtilis
[8]converto
[9]superfluitas
[10]evaporo
[11]repletio

in dura matre vel pia matre, quia tales panniculi sunt duri et *contesti* (contexti) forti *contestura* (contextura). Ideo materia frigida propter grossitiem non potest ingredi (et) hoc dicit Avicenna prima tertii. Alia causa est quia humores frigidi non sunt aequae *mobilles* (molles) sicut calidi, et ideo natura non succurit dolori vel contusioni ita cum frigidis sicut cum calidis.

Tertiam notabile sit istud, quod si intentio medici solum esset in occupatione *solute* (solutionis) continuitatis vel fracturae stante apostemate multa mal accidentia possent consequi, ut coruptio panniculi febris apoplesia (appoplexia) rigor et cetera. Et ideo stante tali apostemate sit occupatio tua in tali cura quae ponitur ab Avicenna principia tertii et non facias hoc cum solis localibus *sicut facit* (ut) simplex *citoycus* sed etiam cum diversionibus.

Quatrum Notabile *sit istud*. Quod in fractura cranei non debet esse occupatio in remotione ossis fracti seu fixi totius, et non queritur in omni fixura et fractura ut accipiatur *os* (eius) totum, quoniam hoc non est possibile, nisi os sit contritum valde et minutum, *iam* tunc enim os est removendum, quia os tale non potest bene nutriri, nec consolidari. Sed considera si os *sit* (est) totaliter perforatum, quia tunc medicus cum abrasione debet usque ad illus latus *penetrare* (pervenire) ut si materia aliqua sub craneo contineatur bene possit egredi. Sed si fractura non sit penetrans medicus non debet tamen abradere; *ymo* (immo) solum usque ad finem *sissure* (scissure) inclusive, et *per* (propter) hoc in *testu dixit* (textu dicit) Avicenna. Frices usquamquo non remaneat de *sissura* (scissura) aliquid, *sed hic adverte quod aliquando est deceptio quia cyroicus putat quod sub craneo non sit aliquid* et tamen latet anguis in herba. Et ideo est considerandum (quid) sit percutiens, (deinde) *et* res cum qua fit percussio, *et hoc facto in isto secundo causu medicina capitalis* (et etiam quid sit subiectum cui est facta percussio, et haec medicina capitalis in hoc casu) est approximanda quae desiccet et uvet in generatione *poris* (porros) *archoydii* (arosebodi) scilicet quando *haec* scissura non penetravit totum os.

Quintum notabile sit istud. Quod in actu prognostico fractura cranei facta abrasione vel abraso osse si panniculus servat situm suum et adventus apostematis non est, aut si est, *et* parvum et adventus saniei adest, si materia ibi continetur, et sanies fit cito, et est bona et laudabilis, [70r] signum est (optimum), quod haec fractura *est* (sit) salubris *plusquam* (potius quam) si panniculus non servat situm suum, et fiat virus, et apostema, et *cum hoc* etiam oportet considerare colorem ossis.

speaks of "hot pus to be cured" and does not mention cold pus. Now the method of cure of hot pus is treated in the first part of three in the chapter *De Carabito*, where he deals with hot pus. Rarely does cold pus develop in the dura mater or pia mater, for such membranes have a hard and firm texture. Cold material, because of its consistency, is not able to penetrate, as Avicenna states in the first part of the third, *in the Chapter De Carabito*. Another reason is that cold humors are not as gentle as hot, and so nature does not soothe pain or contusion with cold as well as with heat.

The third remark. If the intention of the doctor is solely concerned with the break in bone and pus appears, many untoward complications may follow, such as corruption[12] of the membranes, fever, apoplexy, rigor, etc. Should such pus occur, however, the physician should direct his attention to such cures as Avicenna states in the first part of the third applying the cure not to a single location but to diverse areas.

The fourth remark. In skull fractures one should not remove all the loose or impacted fragments, nor should one attempt to grasp all the fragments in every fissure and fracture. This is not possible unless the bone fragments are very comminuted or very small, in which case they should be removed, for such bone can neither derive nourishment nor unite. Consider if the bone is completely pierced, for then the physician ought to debride widely, so that any material contained beneath the skull can easily escape. Similarly, if the fracture does not penetrate, the physician ought not debride, but merely incise to the end of the laceration,[13] concerning which Avicenna states in the text, "rub though you may, nothing is removed from the laceration *and although the surgeon mistakenly believes nothing remains under the bone,* the worm still lurks in the plant". Similarly, the physician must take into account the penetrated bone, the propulsive instrument, and also who it is that received the blow. When the laceration does not completely penetrate the bone, medicines are to be applied which desiccate and benefit the generation of callus.[14]

The fifth remark. With regard to prognosticating accurately in skull fractures after the general debridement has been performed, the following are good omens and favorable [70^r] signs. If the

[12]corruptio
[13]scissure
[14]arosboth

Sextum notabile sit istud, quod cura fracture cranei differt a cura aliarum fracturarum in quatuor. Primo enim quia arosbo*th* quod super os generatur vel inter ossa (sicut cranei) non estaeque durum, sicut illus quod in aliis ossibus generatur. Secundo, quia facta fissura seu fractura non debet esse occupatio medici in restauratione sui; *ymo* (immo) debet ex se remove[ve]ri, sicut dictum est supra, cuius oppostium fit in aliis ossibus, *ymo* (immo) in aliis medicinis facit replasmationem. Tertio, quia in osse capitis non potest fieri ligamentum debitum, sicut in aliis ossibus, et hoc est propter figuram rotundam quam habet caput. Quarto quia dato quod replasmatio ossis fit facta, et per ligaturam, et alia; tamen quia humiditas *per hoc* non est consumpta oportet os removeri. Nam dicit Avicenna quod si humiditas in aliis ossibus retineretur esset necessarium, *quod* (ut) discooperirentur; et ideo *fortius est hic sciendam* (tanto magis hic est fiendum), quia membrum istud est valde nobile. Et propter suam nobilitatem *est* (oportet de ipso) multum *considerandum* (considerare).

Septimum (Aliud) notabile sit istud quod quando medicus habet elevare os debet quartuor considerare. Primo locum convenientem, per quem possit melius et liberius virus egredi, quia locus virulentiae debet esse op[p]ositus per directum *aperture* (loco quem vis aperire). Secundo debet considerare locum faciliorem ad incisionem, quia os *quanto* (quantum) mol[l]ius tantum (melius, quantum ad incisionem ipsius, et) facilius removetur. Tertio tantum debet *removere* (removeri) *quod iterato non oporteat* (de osse quod non oporteat redire), dum in osse est *fixura sive contusio* (scissura sine contusione), quia in contutionibus ubi est contusum et contritum totum (os) in una vice non debet removeri, maxime si est magna quantitas ossis removenda. Sed ratio (prima) *quare* (quod) in s[c]issura primar (sola) vice, illud quod est removendum debet removeri il*l*ico *est* quia si prima vice non removetur tunc est tedium infirmo et astantibus. Secunda quia fluxus materierum ad locum prima vice currit et forte factum est apostema unde panniculi superminent ossi, et *illud* (illus) prohiet abrasionem. Quartro debet locus inquiri qui sit distans *ab* (sub) origine nervorum.

Ottavum (Aliud) notabile sit *istud* (illud, quod Avicenna dicit quod stante fractura cranei tempus remotionis ossis *in estate potest* (debet) esse usque ad septimum diem tempore *in hyeme non* (estibo tempore hyemali vero) usque ad decimum diem. Sed (tamen) dicit Avicenna quanto citius *fiet* tanto melius et longius a timore. (Et

membranes protect their sites and pus does not appear; or if it appears in small amounts accompanied by discharge;[15] and if material is contained at the site and discharge appears rapidly. These kinds of fracture are more healthful than those where the membranes do not cover their site, and slime[16] and pus are generated. Further, one ought consider the color of the bone.

The sixth remark. The cure of cranial fractures differs from the cure of other fractures in four respects. First, with regard to callus tissue which in the skull is generated either above or between bone, the skull callus being softer than callus generated in other bones. Second, the physician should not be concerned with replacing the fragment of fracture or fissure; on the contrary, in skull fractures the fragment must be removed, according to the abovementioned dictum, unlike the situation prevailing in other bones. Furthermore, in other bones, one makes the reconstruction[17] by medicines. Third, one cannot bind the skull like other bones because of the round contour of the cranium. Fourth, from experience we know that even if the contour of the bone be restored through binding, etc., nevertheless the humors are not consumed and it becomes necessary to remove the bone. For Avicenna states that if the humors in any bone be retained, then it is necessary that the bones be distracted, even more so because the skull has great importance. Because of its nobility, great care must be taken with the skull.

Seventh remark. When the physician is compelled to elevate the bone, he must take four matters into consideration. First, a fitting place easily and generously to allow the slime to escape, the location of which ought to be directly over the point he wishes to expose. Second, he ought to consider the most convenient place for the incision. The more pliable the bone, the easier it will be to bring material through the incision and the easier the bone can be removed. Third, in the case of a fracture without bone comminution, one ought to remove as much of the bone as possible in the first attempt, for it is not opportune to return; but where the bone has been battered and bruised, it ought not be removed in one operation, especially if one must remove a great quantity. The reason

[15] sanies
[16] virus
[17] replasmatio

notes) *advertas* quod quatuor sunt casus in quibus non debemus expectare septimum diem, nec decimum *ymo* (immo) vult Avicenna quod fiat in die *secundo* (secunda), vel ad plus in *tertio* (tertia); nisi adsit aliquid congens. Primus casus est, quando constate quod aliqua materia sub craneo continue[a]tur que ad saniem *converteretior* (convertatur) infra illud tempus, que ante eius saniationem debet extrahi. Et quia hoc sepe fit *ideo* non debemus tale tempus expectare, quia circa generationem saniei dolores et febres magis accidunt quam facta sanie. Secundum *casus* (modus) est, quia quando esset aliquod *frustrutum* (frustum) ossis quod pungeret, quia punctio talis esset causa spasmi *et* debemus ipsum cito removere. *Tertius* (Alius) casus est, si esset aliquod foramen per quod materia sub osse ingrederetur. *Quartus* (Alius) casus est, si post fracturam cranei sequeretur infriidatio panniculorum *vel* (et) cerebri vel alterius membri. In hiis enim casibus dicit Avicenna si fuerit *necessaria* (necesse) expectatio, tunc fiat usque ad duos dies aut tres, et si in principio rei oportet ut curetur cum incisione in secundo die.

Nonum (Aliud) notabile sit istud, quod quando nigredo accidit durae matri potet duplici modo contingere. Primo *modo propter unguentum ab extra, approximatum inducens* (per medicinas approximatas inducentes) talem nigredinum. Secundo *modo propter* (per) causam intrinsecam, ut puta, *propter* (per) debilitatem caloris *naturalis sive* innati. Si primo *modo hoc* accidit (per unguentam), tunc cura *perfici debet* (talis sit: Rx: mel cum triplo olei sivi rosati et proiiciatur supra per duas mutationes). Si secondum modo tunc medicus *non debet se impedire* (fugiat a tali curatione); ratio, quia haec nigredo significat *coruptionem* (nigredinem) accidentem [70v] substantile panniculi et *in substantia* (substantiae) cerebri, et hoc est signum mortale et *per consequens mors est propinqua* (mortem propinquam). Sed solum morituri sunt *bresbiteris* (presbyteris) dimittendi.

Decimum (Aliud) notabile sit istud, quod oleum rosatum secundum sententiam Galieni administratur in vulneribus capitis propter timorem eventus apostematis, et propter *sedare dolorem* (sedationem doloris), et inflamationem factum in humoribus et spiritibus, et modo curationis cum ferro. Nam oleum rosatum est doloris mitigativum, et ebulitionis, aut inflammationis *humorum* perfectissime sedativum, et est repercussivum humorum ad locum venientium, et comfortat partes membri circumstantes propter eius stipticitatem quam habet ratione rosarum. Et per consequens

why one removes small rents in one stage is this: if it is not removed in the first operation, then the patient and his nurses are worn out. Second, after the first procedure, a flow of material runs to the site, causing a violent accumulation of pus, whereupon eschar grows over the bone, and this prevents further discharge.[18] Fourth, one ought elect a place distant from the origin of the nerves.

Eighth remark. Avicenna teaches that when a skull fracture occurs, the time for bone removal should be anywhere up to the seventh day in summer, the tenth day in winter. Notwithstanding, Avicenna states, the quicker the better and the less to be feared. Note that there are four instances[19] when one ought not wait for the seventh day nor the tenth day. On the contrary, Avicenna recommends the second day, or, unless contraindicated, the third day at the latest. The first instance is when one has established that material is present beneath the skull which threatens to be converted into discharge. Before this happens, and it happens often, the material should be removed. One does not await the stated time, because pain and fever occur with the generation of discharge[15] more than after it has been generated. The second instance is when a fragment of bone penetrates,[20] for such punctures[21] are the cause of spasm and should be quickly removed. The third instance is when bone defects[22] are present through which material enters beneath the bone. The fourth instance occurs when, after skull fracture, rents[23] occur in the membranes, the cerebrum or any other structure. In all these instances Avicenna states that if one must wait, perform the operation in the early stages before the second or third day. If one must cure by incising,[24] then incise on the second day.

Ninth remark. When black discharge[25] occurs in the dura mater, it can happen in two ways: first, by the application of the medicines which cause this black discharge; second, from intrinsic causes as, for example, through the breakdown of the body's heat. If the first occur because of ointments, then its remedy is this. Rx:

---

[18]abrasio
[19]casus
[20]pungere
[21]punctio
[22]foramen
[23]infrindatio
[24]incisio
[25]nigredo

oleum rosatum in principio et augmento in fracturis capitis et eius percussionibus est summa medicina, medicinarum et maxime est prohibitivum eventus apostematis.

Undecim notabile sit istud (Aliud sit notabile), quod vinum contussum cum oleo rosato et panno lini *inbibito et* in percussionibus capitis supra posito dat magnum iuvamentum, (et) etiam ex parte vini stiptici gratia exiccationis que competit vulneri, et sua stipticitate adivuat ad prohibendum fluxum humorum ad locum, sed (et) confert ratione panni duplicati vel triplicati in tali oleo rosato et vino ut diutius tale medicamen in panno illo retineatur.

III

Capitulum tertium quod est exemplum.

Venit ad me cum auxilio divinae trinitatis quidam rusticus et nomine gacabinus cum uno suo nepote quod quandam fuit vulneratus tribus vulneribus et cum uno cultello quorum unum vulnus erat in intestino colon et exivit pro tunc quando primo vidi stercus de vulnere illo et erat in illo situ ubi est revolutio renis sinistri. Aliud vulnus erat in casso et penetrabat, signum fuit quod aer exiens de illo vulnere extinxit ignem unius candelae magne accense. Aliud vulnus erat in splene quem vidi, et exibat a vulnere sanguis niger melancolicus et tale vulnus erat sub costis mendosis in parte sinistra, quae omnia vulnera in illo suo nepote iam liberaveram. Et de vulnere intestini exivit magnus lumbricus quasi in fine consolidationis, quem lumbricum extrassi de vulnere cum manibus meis.

Honey with triple oil or rose oil. Cover the area with two different applications. If the second situation has occurred, then the physician may as well abandon hope for a cure, for this black substance signifies corruption [70v] in the membranes and in the brain substance. This is a fatal sign, indicating that death is near. But only the moribund should be handed over to the priests.

Tenth remark. Rose oil, following Galen's opinion, should be administered in head wounds when there is danger of pus, and because of its ability to comfort pain and inflammation generated in the humors and spirits. It is also used as an adjuvant to the cure by iron cautery. Rose oil eases pain. It is a most wonderful sedative for blistering and inflammation. It prevents the humors from coming to the site and comforts the surrounding structures through its styptic action, which is due to the roses. Rose oil, then, is an excellent medicine for skull fractures and concussion[26] in the incipient stage and in the stage of augmentation, chiefly because it prevents the appearance of pus.

Eleventh remark. If a linen dressing is impregnated with a mixture of rose oil and wine and the dressing placed above the injured head, this affords much relief, even serving as a styptic wine for drying.[27] All this is beneficial[28] to wounds. Further, the styptic properties assist in preventing the flow of humors to the site. But soak the dressing two or three times in this oil and wine mixture that it may be retained longer on the dressing.

Chapter III

Section III, wherein is contained a Case Report.

With the help of the Divine Trinity, a certain peasant named Gacabinus came to me in the company of his nephew, who, on one occasion, had been wounded in three places with a knife. The first wound had been in the colon at the hepatic flexure and when I first saw it, feces issued from the wound. The second wound had penetrated into the depths, as evidenced by the fact that air escaping from that wound extinguished the flame of a large, lighted candle. The third wound had been in the spleen which I saw. Black

[26]percussio
[27]exiccatio
[28]completo

Dixit itaque dictum Gacabinus cuius filius adhuc iam de fractura cranei habui in cura et liberavi filius meus Pasqualinus percussit confratre istius quem tu a morte sanasti quemdam iuvenem portatorem cum uno spito de cinglario et auriculum spiti fixit in capite modicum lateraliter et parum distans a commissura coronali per unam unguem infra. Sed duo alii homines qui erant secum iuraverunt mihi quod viderunt ex illa hora cum sanguine exire de substantia cerebri quando posuerunt albumenae ovi hoc modo certe volui credere. Sed recordans me ex verbis Galieni septem particula afforismorum anforismo illo. Vesuum iscisam et in comment dicit Galienus de cerebro incisionem quoque cerebri multotiens vidi sanari. Semel enim vidi in intabia civitate Sammaria quandam magne et concave incisum cerebrum habere et tamen mortem evadere quod contingit rarissme.

Item Renaldus de Villanova in sua practica et in tertio tractatu dicit hoc idem audivisse a pertissimis ciroicis de substantia cerebri exire et a morte egrotantes evadere. Sed hoc vidi oculis meis de substantis medulari iterum in hoc egro exire quem curavi solus sine alio consilio in presentia multorum doctorum et scolarium paduanorum quos precibus meis et caritate mecum ducebam ut viderent possibilitatem nature scilicet separationem manifestam et amplam per duos digitos per ventriculi anterioris in quo ymaginativa [71[r]] *perficitur a separatione medii ventriculi in quo cogitatio sive ratio perficitur. Tertius ventriculus posterior ubi fiat retentiva sive virtus tanta tezaurizativae non fuit pro tunc mihi ad oculum in tali homine vivo. Omnes iste tres virtutes fuerunt semper sicut sane et sine aliquo accidente omnibus accidentibus numeratis solentibus apparere in huiusmodi dispositionibus sicut vomitus Sincopis Singultus spasmus alienatio mentis febres et epilepsia. Virtus nutritiva animalis vitalis fuerunt semper sicut sanae usque ad trigesimaquarta diem in qua die supervenit quinque parosismis epilepsie cum magno sudore et febre continua et hoc fuit a causa primitive scilicet a potatione vini montani me nesciente. Sed verum est quod illa dies fuit etiam dies cretica salubris et radicativa secundum quod numeravi per computacionem dierum medicinalium creticorum sed transacta illa die remansit debilitas in virtute motiva ex parte contraria pedis et manus. Sed modus qualiter ego processi ipsum curando tam practice quam teorice inferius narrabo.*

bilious blood escaped from the wound. The last wound was located under the floating rib on the left. All of his nephew's wounds I had cured. Moreover, at the end of the healing process, there had issued forth from the intestinal injury a large worm, which I removed from the wound with my hands.

And so this man, Gacabinus, whose son I had already treated and cured of a fractured skull said, "My son, Pasqualinus, the brother of a boy you saved from death, struck a certain porter with a boar spear, driving the tip into his head, a short distance lateral to and one finger below the coronal commissure. The other two men who were with him swore to me, because they witnessed it, that when they applied egg albumen, blood spurted out, together with brain substance." Although I found this hard to believe, I recalled the words of Galen in the seventh aphorism, "Vesunam incisam", in which he states concerning the brain, "I have seen incisions into the brain often heal, for on one occasion in Intabia [Ionia?], a city of Sammaria, I saw a certain person escape death who had a huge concave incision of the cerebrum. This rarely occurs."

Item. Renaldus de Villanova, in the third tractate of his Practica, states the following. Item: "I have heard from experienced surgeons of the patient surviving, despite the loss of cerebral substance, a rare occurrence." Moreover, with my own eyes I have seen the herniation of grey matter, which condition I cured without other assistance in the presence of many doctors and scholars of Padua, whom I enticed there with prayers and charity, that they may witness the possibilities of nature, namely a wide apparent separation of the first anterior ventricle where imagination [71^{r}] *is perfected, two finger-breadths from the middle ventricle, where cogitation or reasoning occurs. The posterior third ventricle where retention or memory abides, was never before seen by me in a living man. All these three faculties continued to remain healthy without involvement by any of the numerous usual accidents presenting as the following symptoms, i.e., vomiting, syncope, singultus, spasm, irrationality, fever, and epilepsy. The nutritive, animal and vital faculties remained normal until the thirty-fourth day, at which time five epileptic fits occurred, accompanied by profuse sweating and persistent fever. These resulted from a primitive cause, namely, the patient drank mountain wine without my knowledge. Moreover, this day was numbered a critical, healthy and influential time, according to my computations of the critical days of medicine. At the end of the day, weakness in the motor faculties remained because of contraries of the feet and hand. The practical and theoretical methods with which I proceeded to remedy this state of affairs, I shall relate below.*

IV

Sequitur Capitulum Quartum et Universale in Fracturis Capitis et Theoricum.

Hoc est capitulum universali et theorecum de vulneribus et fracturis capitis. Sed ut plenam doctrinam de vulneribus et fracturis capitis habeas lege libros quos ego transcursi ut alios quod fuerunt meo tempore laude notati ut princeps medicorum. Primus scilicet scalapius a primo medicinae inventor et anasagorus de secta empiricorum et Viaticus de secta thesilicorum. Et ypocras verus claviger omnium egritudinum cum galieno et avicenna et conciliatore et cum continente secta omnium virtutum sibelium medicinalium. Alii itaque tubatores in hac facultate sicut Guglielmus de Vergnana alius gordensis de pedemontium Guidonus Faba Gulielmus de placenta Brunus longoburgensis de padua Teodricus de cervia episcopus in hac facultate dignus Renaldus de villa nove sive Floriquerus et rugerius cum alafranco atque alberto et Xgellate cum trusano atque peritissimo Serapione cum albucasi in hac sciencia ad oculum in aliquibus egritudinibus valde confusi. (Sequitur de fracturis cranei in universali.

Hoc est capitulum universale theoricum de vulneribus et fracturis capitis, sed ut plenam doctrinam de vulneribus et fracturis capitis habeas lege libros qui sunt a me pluries nominati, et de primis medicinae inventoribus fuit Esculapius et Anaxagoras de secta Empicorum, et Viaticus de secta Thesilicorum. Et Hypocras verus primus omnium egritudinum cum Galieno et Avicenna et Conciliator. Aliiquam Tubatores sicut Glummus Gulielmus de Vergnaza. Lilius gordensis. Franciscus de Pedemonte. Guidonus faba, Guilelmus de Placentia. Et magister Betinus de Rabis de Parma qui optime dixit in hac arte. Brunus seu Bernucius Parmemsis cum peritissimo Serapione, atque Albucasi manifest in aliquibus egritudinibus valde confusi) sed ad intellectum valde provecti. *Quare* (quia) fides *itaque* non est conclusive cuilibet narranti adhibenda, nisi *ex* (id) experimento vel ratione *clare notescat* (manifesta clarefiat). Fractura cranei cum sit aliis ossibus periculosior et *difficilisima quo* (difficilior) ad curandum *patentur species fracturarum optime oportet a medico bene considerare* (oportet eius species considerare). Nam fractura aliquando fit cum ense, aliquando *fit* cum lapide, aliquando (cum) ligno, *sive* (aliquando cum) bac(c)ulo et *similia contundentia* (similibus contundentibus). Fractura aut est parva aut (est) magna, et ad oculum saepe occulta. Hoc est quando multotiens accidit ut *findatur* (scindatur) craneum et non *findatur*

Chapter IV

A general chapter on the theory of skull fractures.

This is the theoretical section concerning wounds and fractures of the head. That you may have a complete understanding of wounds and fractures of the head, read the works which I frequently note. The discoverers of the first medicines were Esculapius and Anaxagoras of the sect of Empiricus; Viaticus, of the sect of Thesily; and Hippocrates, truly the first to describe all illnesses, as well as Galen, Avicenna, the Conciliator, and the related sects of all the meritorious sibyline medicines. Other leaders in this faculty are Glummus de Vergnoza; Lilius Gordensis of Pedmont; Brunus Longoburgo of Padua; Theodoricus of Cervia, respected leader in this faculty; Renaldus of Villanova; Florigerus; Rugerius; Alafrancus; Albertus; Anagellatus; Trusiano Franciscus of Pedmont; Guidonus Faba; Guilemus de Placentia; Master Bertinus de Rabis of Parma; the well informed Serapione; and Abucase, who, in the observation of some diseases displayed great confusion, but who has a most accomplished intellect. Trust incompletely anything cited as an authority unless it be explained by experiment or by reason. Inasmuch as skull fractures are, compared to other bone fractures, more dangerous and difficult to cure, one might best consider their classification. Fractures are sometimes caused by sword, rock, club, sticks and other similar weapons.[29] Fractures can be either small or large and hidden from the eye. It often happens that the skull is fractured, although the skin is not scratched, as Avicenna tells us in the fourth section of four in the section *De Fractura Cranei*.

Item. Fractures are sometimes associated with large wounds, other times with small wounds. At times only part of the bone is removed in the fracture. Sometimes when the skull is pierced by a weapon and other similar objects, the skull can be perforated. This situation here is more dangerous than in other bones. At times the fracture will appear small to the eye, yet be deep in the bone. Sometimes a small linear fracture[30] or a nick[31] occurs, such as to be undiscernible to the naked eye unless some rash experiment[32] be

[29]contendentes
[30]fractura capilaris
[31]fractura rimularis
[32]experiment incaustro

(scindatur) cutis, ut tangit Avicenna *quarta* (quinta) *quartem* (quarti) et in capitulo de fractura cranei.

Item fractura aliquando est cum vulnere magno, aliquando cum vulnere parvo. Sed in fractura aliquando pars ossis removetur, aliquando craneum *perforatur* (perforamus), quod aliis ossibus est *sustectior et periculosior ut quando hoc* (magis suspectum ut periculosum ut quandoque) contingit *cutelli missille sagipta* (ipsum perforari cum telo sagitta), et similibus. *Quoniam* aliquando *vulnus appareatur* ad oculum apparebit parvum, et profunditas *fracturae celantur* (in osse) erit magna. Aliquando fit in osse fractura rimularis *vel* (sive) capillaris, taliter quod solor visu non potest dis(c)erni, nisi cum experimento *enclaustri* (incaustri), et sunt quandoque in craneo *plicatura* (plicature) ut in pueris, et in cranei molli, quod *consuevit fieri et* (consuivit accidere pueris), maxime quando cadunt de alto. Aliquando contingit caput ledi in una parte et os ipsius *cranei* frangi in alia, quoniam ossa cranei comparantur vitro *et hoc est* (ob hoc, et ideo) quia sunt differentissima in curando ab aliis ossibus aliorum membrorum. Sed *solers* (prudens) medicus, *sicut prudens* debet itaque has omnes species fracturarum per *inquistionem contentis et ingenii laborantis inquiri* (ingenium inquirere), quoniam ingenium et cautela sine scientia saepe facit hominem magnum philosophum (reputari).

Nam *de* (in) lesione cranei, et panniculorum [71[v]] cerebri non possumus de *liberatione patientis sperare* (salute infirmi iudicare) et maxime si egrotantem videris se desere a *cura* (spe) salutis; quoniam tales morituri ex motione astrorum movebunt linguam *quasi in* (ex) omni tua visitatione cum petieris de sanitate eorum bene vel male de se prognosticando veritatem dicent, (quia dicent ego moriar.) Spes ergo nostra *ponenda est cum de talibus qui artificio cirurgie curari volunt non multum sperandum sit nisi in solo deo et natura que ab ipso est*. (In talibus qui artificio cyrurgiae curari non possunt ponenda est in deo; et facere quicquid potes, quia aliquando morituros vivere vidi). Medicus qui huiusmodi talem *habere* (habet) in *habere* cura spem necesse est et salutem semper infirmo permictere et parentibus suis, *alibi* (deinde) periculum mortis *de egro* narrare, ne *stolidus vulgus de te et contra te deveniat ad cloquendum et dehonestandum*. (Stolidi vulgares tibi possint detractare), et si certus fueris et videbis *talem casum* (tali casui) imminere periculum, *te* (tu) et dic infirmo. O *frater mi* (amice mi) *te ordinare* (ordina) testamentum et confiteri deo *peccata tua* (tuorum peccatorum) *quid* (quia) erit

employed. Sometimes the fracture takes the form of plication[33] of the bone, as in children, especially when they fall from heights, and in people with soft heads. Sometimes the head is hit in one place and the bone itself fractures in another, for the bones of the skull are comparable to glass and they differ in their cure from other bones. The prudent physician ought to inquire into all these classifications with intelligence, for intelligence and caution, even without knowledge, often makes a man renowned as a great philosopher.

In lesions[34] of the membranes of the head and brain, [71^v] we are not able to determine the health of the patient, and less so when one sees that the patient has abandoned hope for recovery. Such dying persons move their tongues under the influence of the motion of the stars and, foreseeing the truth, say during his visits when the physician seeks to ascertain whether their health be good or bad, "I will die." The hope, then, in those who cannot be cured with surgery is to be placed in God; yet, do as much as you can for them, for sometimes I have seen these moribund survive. The physician who treats such patients must have faith, ever holding out hope of recovery to the patient and his family. Later, however, if he is certain of the outcome and sees such conditions as forebode danger, he must, lest the stupid criticize and calumniate him, inform the patient of the peril of death. He must say to the patient, "Oh, my friend, compose your testament and confess your sins to God, which will be very helpful to me and beneficial for the cure, healing your wounds the more quickly, for your mind will be at peace and your humors cleansed of strange fancies."[35]

Similarly, my son, entrusted with the cure of these sick people, while hoping in God and nature, you ought to administer the needs of nature with deception; and give the sick all they desire. But in dangerous illnesses taste and retaste without deception anything you intend to administer, for if it works badly from the standpoint of nature, and endangers the physician, it will quickly cause the patient's destruction.

The following concerns the cure of skull fractures.

Diligent physicians always regard as serious the treatment of

---

[33]plicatura
[34]lesio
[35]ab extraneis imaginationibus

mihi valde *utile* (commodum et iocundum), pro cura *tua* et *cito* sanabitur tuum vulnus, quia tua mens erit pacifica et humores tui erunt magis ab extraneis *ymaginationibus* (imaginationibus) depurati.

Ideo tu *filii* (amice) qui talem infirmum habes in cura in deo, et natura sperando diligenter et sagaciter debes naturae necessaria sine fallicia administrare (scilicet dare egrotis omnia quae volunt). *Primo ergo glutias et deglutias et sine inducia in forti egritudinem antequam aliquod agas quoniam male agere a natura et peius a te medico crede absque dubio quod vita illius destructionis eris causa.*

Sequitur Capitulum de curatione fracturarum ossis capitis et hoc in universali.

Curatio vulnerum sive fracturam ossis capitis semper a medico diligentissime est consideranda tanquam gravis (et) suspecta *et periculosa* egritudo. Primo ergo oportet *ut universalia non obliviscaris* (ne obliviscaris universalia) ut *per ea* valeas ad paticularia operari. Universalia sunt sicut flebotomia evacuationes per solventia, (et) diversiones per ventosas, et per curas et clisteria *qualiter lege et per lege bene nostros precessores si vis scire quomodo qualiter et quando ista debeant fieri quam hic intendo quod celum penetret brevis oratio*.

Porro in hoc casu de fractura cranei, et in quam pluribus aliis, quos ego sanavi, cum inueniebam lunam *circumcirca* (circa) combustionem consistere semper inveni visione manifesta et mensurabili cerebrum a craneo per unum digitum cum panniculis lateraliter esse plus quam depressum, putavi aut (quod) hoc *esset* (accidisset) ex tempore cordis egrotantis quando percussus fuit, *propter territum* aut quod luna propter dominium humiditatum diminuendo in tali tempore *talis fecisset elongatio* (diminuisset, et fecisset hanc dilatationem), tunc affirmavi illud caput humidum non esse a praedominio superfluvum, et si cum magna speculatione *curando et dirigendo* (in evacuatione et digestione) pro tunc me non oportebat uti, et hoc si aer cibus et potus, motus et quies, *sompnus* (somnus) et vigilia, inanitio et repletio, et accidentia animae erant illi egro debito modo bene applicata; et si tertia virtus in suo robore *bene* perseverabat semper salutem *faciebam* (reddidi) cuilibet egrotanti. Si autem *suspicasse posse* (aliquid coniectasset) aliquid mali, *accidere* quod esset distructio *naturarum* (naturalium et spiritualium) animalium, vitalium *et naturalium* illud semper *ante* rectificare conabar, quo facto salus et vita (illi egrotanti) in quadragenta diebus illi

wounds or fractures of the bones of the head and view the outcome of such illness as uncertain. Consider first, if you have forgotten anything of value in the particular task, the useful things, being phlebotomy and evacuation[36] by solvents,[37] etc., cupping,[38] cures and clysteries.[39] *Read and reread our predictions if you want to know the how and whys, for the heavens bless a short account.*

Moreover, in the cases of fractured skulls and other conditions which I cure, when I see a burning around the moon, I always establish with clear and measurable observation that the distance from the brain and the membranes is one finger below the skull defect. In my opinion, however, this happened either because of fear in the heart of the patient at the time he sustained the blow or because the moon with its power over moisture, lessened and created this dilatation by lessening the moisture at this time. Then, I affirmed that that moist heat is not flowing over from the influence of that dominance; I am not obliged to use extensive observation about evacuation and digestion[40] if good food and drink, motion and quiet, sleep and awakeness, dieting[41] and plethora[42] and the things proper to the soul are correctly administered to the patient in due measure. If the third virtue persists in its robustness, health will always return to whoever is ill. If, however, anything untoward is applied which destroys nature or spiritual living creatures, this I always attempt to rectify. This done, health and life return to the patient in the fortieth day of the illness. I have even seen one peasant, part of whose medulla was removed, who is at present healthy.

(Note, therefore, friends) *that in this condition, first, wine and air are to be similarly avoided until the patient is well. These contraries are always inimical.* Second, the patient should drink only boiled water and sugar and he must remain in a quiet room without fresh air. If it is cold, insure that the room is continuously heated with a good fire. His diet should consist of pancakes[43] with yolk of chicken egg

[36] evacuatio
[37] solventio
[38] ventosis
[39] clisteria
[40] digestio
[41] initio
[42] repletio
[43] panata

egrotanti *infallabiliter erit sospes (reddebatur). Venio ergo filii mi ad causum arduum quem tibi promisi. Nam qui potest fracturam magnam cranei sanare quanto brevius erit illi medico sanare per naturam. Huic informo scilicet de quo remota fuit de substantia medulari cerebri. Primo dixi nota quod duo contraria te semper sunt inimici scilicet vinum et aer quare ab eis fuge si vis habere salutem. Secundo*. (Et semel habui unum rusticum qui erat remota pars medullaris cerebri qui est sanatus.

Nota ergo amice quod in hoc casu duae regulae sunt observande, ut infirmus primum non bibat, nisi) aquam *cottam* (coctam) cum *zucero* (zucharo) *bibe* et (ut stet) in camera latebrosa, id est, sine luciditate aeris, *semper permane*. (Et) si frigus sit *fit* (fac ut) in *illo talamo* (illa camera) continue ardeat ignis (magnus). Cibus (suus) sit panata cum uno vitello pulli aut *cum* brodio pulli sine sale, (quoniam nihil est magis pestiferum, et quod magis inducat lapidem in vesica quam sal), saltem in prima *edomada* (hebdomada), postea *comede* (comedat) aliquam *partem* (particellam) pulli, et farrum et risum cum lacte, seminum communium, [72^r] et non *comedas* (comedat) masticabilia in his primis temporibus, quia fortis masticatio est causa commotionis materiarum ad locum lesum, propter colligantiam lacertorum *et* panniculorum cum mandibula inferior quae mandibula habet motum voluntarium. In *tertia procedabam* (Interea) secundum quod mihi ostendebat praeco, *id est pulsus* qui nunqum fallit, *experto musico* (expertum musicum), hoc dico, quia debes sciri quod in pulsu reperitur natura musicae, quoniam per adiunctionem sonorum, id est motuum, cognoscuntur eorum proportionalitates, et sic per medicum expertum potest cognosci *patenter vitam egrotantis esse propinquam vel remotam* (vita egrotantis propinqua aut remota) termino moritis.

Item *aspiciebat* (aspice) urinam quae est *nuctius* (nuncius) quatuor qualitatum primarum existentium in vasis servientibus toti corpori *viventi. Et sic tamquam comitus velum dirigebam quocumque citius potui versus portum salutis.*

Tertio dixi (Secundo dic) semper (egro) sta in lecto, ne aliquis motus sit causa *ut* febris *superveniat* (supervenientis) cum in omni motu *fit* (sit) calefactio, et cum omnis febris tam naturaliter quam effective sit calida. Ergo quietus stet infirmus et permaneat quantum potest sine motu.

Quatro *dixi* (die dic informo) si *potes* (potest) domire *ad tuum bene placitum* (quiete, et sicut consuevisti) de nocte, cum somnus sit maxime de vigorantibus virtutem et cum de prosternentibus

or unsalted chicken broth. Nothing is more harmful[44] and more productive of bladder stone than salt, at least during the first week. Afterwards, he may eat a small piece of chicken, grain, rice with milk and ordinary seeded grain. [72^r] Do not let him eat things that must be chewed at this early stage, for vigorous mastication causes the movement of material to the site of the lesion, the mandible having voluntary motion through the connection of the ligaments[45] of the membranes with the mandible below. In the third day, I proceed according to the signal which I perceive in the pulse, for it never deceives an experienced musician. I say this, since you should know that the nature of music is found in the pulse and from the rhythm[46] (i.e., movement), their proportions can be interpreted, and the informed physician can thereby discern whether the life of the patient be far or near the time of death.

Item. Examine the urine, which is the messenger[47] of the four primary qualities in the vessels serving the entire living body. Thus, like a captain, I direct sail as quickly as possible to the port of health.

Third, always have the patient stay in bed, lest motion of any kind be the cause of supervening fever. Heat is generated by all motion, and every fever generates warmth, both by its nature and in its side effects. The patient, therefore, must be quiet and immobile, as much as possible.

Fourth, ask the patient to sleep quietly as is his wont at night, since sleep is the greatest promoter of the qualities of vigor, while restlessness, pain, and fever are its destroyers, all of which I hope to spare him.

Fifth, on the seventh day I apply clysters, cures or suppositories, or I administer syrup[48] with the appropriate digestive material, followed by cinnamon,[49] date electuary[50] or a general electuary to promote the passage of gas.

Sixth, I bid the patient insure that his mind be ever happy and without evil thoughts and tell him soothing and humorous things in

---

[44]persiferum
[45]lacertus
[46]adjuctio
[47]nuncius
[48]syrupos
[49]cassia
[50]diafinicone

maxime (valde)sit vigilia; dolor et feter, *ergo hiis omnibus malis abicere ab informo canonice intendebam. Vigilie Filonium aliqua reges aliqua pillas somponiferas huiusmodi similter post cenam dabam* (et hec omnia ab informo abiicere intendebam).

Quinto aliquando clisteria aut curam aut *sopostam, i.e.* suppositoria faciebam saepissime imponi, aut syrupos cum digestione appropriateae materiae dabam postea cum cassia, aut disfinicone (aut) electario indo *et huiusmodi* venetrem solvebam.

Sexto dixi fac quod tua mens semper stet *hilaris* (ylaris) et sine aliqua mala cogitatione, *quare dicebam* (et dic egrotanti quando) ipsum *medendo semper* (curas) rem placabilem et iocosam. Sed cum haec egritudo tam *occulum* (intellectum) quam ad *intellectum sit* (occulum fuit) mihi manifesta, scias quod raro aliquem excoriavi, dummodo via sive cerebrum (haberet) respiraculum. Ratio: natura omnia agit. Medicus vero illam credendo (credens illam) iuvare (intendit vel) impedit. Sed *si pur* (tantum) excoriabam (et) hoc faciebam cum moicula paulatine sublevando pellem *a craneo* cum *almocatim* (almocati) in duabus visitationibus, in tres visitatione *novacula* (cum moicula) furtive incidebam, et cum albumine ovi fluxus sanguinis, si expediebat restringebam. Ultra hoc cum stuellis stupeis, quia *frigi* (frigidi) sunt madefactis in oleo rosato, calido et expressis mutabam et cum illis leviter labia excoriata *triangulariter* (triangulata) vel *quadrangulariter* (quadrangulata) elevabam, et sic parum inferebam egro nocumentum, si bene *intellexistis me et habeas* (me intellexisti habeas) modum.

Ulterius ut supra notavi, *quod* (et) si aliquod (os) erat (vel erit) elevandum illud non *movebam vi quoniam ossa* (extrahebam, quia os) numquam *violenter debenta medico extrahi* (a medico violenter extrahi debet) nisi pungat, aut nocumentum velaminibus et cerebro faciat. Patio quia dolor est cause attractionis *humoris* (humorum) ad locum, *et* facit in cerebro, aut in panniculo apostema, sive *spasmus accidet* (spasmum accidere) et sic in futuro tu male operando, et cum dolore egri mortis eris causa; et sic sequetur cum *tuo* illato dolore novissimus error *et* prior priore. (Et) Semper medicina *in fractura cranei sive* capitis debet esse *ab ygne* (sub igne) calefacta, et *per* (propter) hoc semper habe *habui tegulam calefactum* (calefactivum textum) supra caput infirmi, *ipsum* mutando, ne frigus *extrinsecus adveniat* (veniret) velaminibus cerebri. *Postquam* (Postea) vero removi ossa si putabam aliquid remansisse de dolore.

Rx: (Recipiebam) vitellum ovi conquassatum cum oleo rosato calido et stuellis *intrati* (intinctis) in hoc medicamine vulnus *replebam*

the course of treatment. But since this disease is revealed to me as much by the mind as by the eye, be advised that rarely do I debride[51] as long as the passageway of the brain is respiring. The reason: nature takes care of everything. The physician, in truth, believing to help, threatens or hinders. But when I must debride, I perform this with a *moicula*, elevating the skin from the skull by degrees with almon in the course of two visits. During the third visit, I furtively incise with the *moicula,* applying egg white, if necessary, to repress the flow of blood. Further, I use a drain stupe cooled and rinsed in rose oil, and gently raise the triangular or quadrangular excoriated edges of the wound. This causes only minimal trauma to the patient if I have done my work well.

Furthermore, as noted above, if any bone has been or will be elevated, it must not be removed, for the bone ought never to be violently removed by the physician unless it penetrates or does harm to the membrane[52] or brain. The reason: pain causes the attraction of the humors to the site, inducing pus or spasm in the brain or membranes. From a poor operation and the production of pain in the patient, one might cause his death. As a result of the pain, therefore, additional error follows in succession. The medicines for the head should always be heated under fire and must always be kept warm on the patient's head through frequent changes, lest external cold injure the covering of the brain. Afterwards, to be sure, I remove the bone if I think that anything remains which can cause pain.

Rx: Soak a stupe in yolk of egg, mixed with hot rose oil. Insert it into the wound, applying around it hot rose oil.

Item. Sometime I merely moisten the drain in hot rose oil, and, squeezing out the excess, I lay the drain somewhere in the wound and observe discharge generating in the wick. Before doing this, however, I first cut the hair over the drain and, so that the medicament may better adhere to the part of the lesion, I apply our ointment, which has a nice white consistency, diffusing to the bulging flesh a pleasant odor. It works wondrously [72^{v}] in the brain by divine qualities. The name of ointment of resin of pine, given to us by the Conciliator, is of great value in comforting the brain and in effectively reducing pain by withdrawing[53] the discharge from

[51]excorio
[52]velaminibus
[53]exicatio

(implebam), et circumcirca, cum oleo rosato calido vulnus inungebam.

Item aliquando solum madefaciebam stuellos *cum solo* (in oleo) rosato calido, et *aliquando* expressis ab ipso oleo vulnus implebam usquequo in vulnere, et in stuellis saniem videbam fieri. Sed supra stuellos prius incisis capillis, ut medicamina *capita sive* illi parti lese melius adherent, ponebam tale nostrum unguentum, quod habet *colorem album ad* (formam albam et)*formam* pulchram. Et carunculis mam[m]illaribus facit in redolendo suavem odorem, et agit in cerebro miraculose [72v] qualitatem divinam, et vocatur unguentum de resine pini relatum ad *conciliationem* (conciliatore) quod unguentum est tante dignitatis in comfortando cerebrum et *vehementer facientem* (in faciendo) vehementer quiescere dolorem *et* ex*s*iccando superfluitatem de sub osse, absque abrasione et detectione ipsius ossis, *quod* (et) est mirum et incredibile *se* (et) administratur, maxime post incisionem fracti et eradicationem sec[a]ti et extractionem fracturae, tot et tanta *inducit* (inducat) bona *et* occulta *ut expertus quid esset* (que expertus fui, ut esset) longum narrare. Attamen non est mirandum secundum sententiam Galieni *dicendo* (dicentis) quod *complexio* (compositio) ossis et panniculi est (humida et) sicca.

Unguentum autem est tale (in principio) Rx: resina[e] pini mollis et albe unc. ii; olei rosati unc. i; gummi elemi unc. ss; cere albae quod sufficit. Fiat unguentum malaxatum cum vino montano, et istud unguentum per malaxationem *fiet* (fit) magis album.

Item supra istud unguentum *meum* mirabile ponebam *istud meum* tale emplastrum, quod est comfortativum cerebri mirabiliter et in pauco tempore.

Emplastrum *autem* est tale. Rx: calamenti, florum camomille, melliloti, sticados arabici, foliorum lauri assari, bet*h*onicae, matris silvae ana M. i; maiorane, serpili[i] ana M. ss; farine ordei M. i; olei rosati unc. iii; olei camomellini unc. ii; fiat emplastrum et adde in fine decoctionis *croci* scrup ii; quoniam *crocis* (crocum ortulanum) ingreditur in omni sedatione doloris, ut tangit Avicenna decima tertii in (capitulo) de passionibus spiritualium. Sed quando vulnus penetrabat, quandoque craneum et facta digestione *ab* (cum) oleo rosato exinde *antea* (ad valutem) continuo usque ad finem curae, ponebam in vulnere mel rosatum solum, et non oleum rosatum cum melle, sicut faciunt *quasi* (communiter) omnes *praticantes* (isti barbitonsores). Nam hunc malum errorem *sepe* audivi *commicti*

under the bone so that you do not have to debride or uncover[54] the bone itself. Its action is wonderful and incredible, especially when expressly administered after the incision has been made and after the cut part has been rooted out and the fracture fragments extracted. So many and so wonderful the secrets produced by this could be related by the experienced physician that it would take long to enumerate; nevertheless, the aforementioned is not surprising and is in accordance with the words of Galen who teaches that the composition of the bone and membranes is humid and dry.

This is the ointment used in the beginning of the illness. Rx: soft white resin of pine 2 ounces; oil of roses 1 ounce; gum of myrrh half an ounce; white wax of sufficient quantity. Make an ointment and mix with mountain wine, the ointment from the admixture is whiter. Item. Over this wonderful ointment I place this plaster, which quickly soothes the brain in wondrous fashion.

This is the plaster. Rx: Calamenth, flowers of camomile, meliot, lavender, flowers of laurel, asarabacca, betony, mater sylvia of each 1 fistful; majory, wild thyme of each half a fistful; barley meal 1 fistful; oil of roses 3 ounces; oil of camomile 2 ounces. Make a plaster and add saffron 2 scruples. Boiled saffron soothes pain, as Avicenna teaches in the tenth part of three, the section *De Passionibus Spiritualum*. But when the wound penetrates to the skull and digestion has been performed with rose oil, then, until health is regained at the end of the cure, I continue placing in the wound only red honey—not rose oil with honey as the barbers[55] are wont to do. I have heard this grievous error committed in patients with fractured skulls. Some physicians who treated them continue to apply rose oil, resulting—so I hear—in death. The reason: Avicenna, in the beginning of the third in the section *De Incisione et Plaga*, cites Galen, saying that membranes and bone have a dry composition.[56] I continue with the plasters until I think the brain has taken on a good constitution, effecting this by vigorous digestion. I have even had the following situation occur twice in two weeks. The patient's head did not require perforation, neither by the iron trepan nor by the perforating trepan.[57] *The method whereby this procedure, when required, should be performed is universally recounted*

[54]detectio
[55]barbitonsores
[56]sicce complexiones
[57]trepano ferrino neque trepano perforatoris

(committi) et (aliquando) quam plures egrotantes de fractura cranei *meo tempore* existentes *in* manibus aliquorum medicorum et hac assidua perseveratione olei rosati *scio mori* (audivi mortuos). Ratio quia *Avicenna principia tertii in capitulo de incisione et plaga dicit auctoritate Galieni in de complexionibus quia* (panniculus est siccae complexionis, et etiam compositio ossis) *complexio ossis et panniculi est sicca*. Sed cum emplastro tandium procedebam donec cerebrum putabam *optimum* (bonam) fortitudinem assumpsisse cum digestionis vigoramento, et *in hoc* (hunc) casu(m) *fuit* (habuibis) in duabus [h]ebdomadis. Craneum huius egri non oportuit cum *tripano* (trepano) ser[r]ino neque trepano perforatorio perforari. *Modus qualiter debeat fieri si necesse unquam fuerit ab aliis auctoribus adisce quare hic taceo quoniam non fuit causa necessitatis.*

In foramine vero huius cranei *egri* nullum aliud abstersivum posui, nisi mel rosatum simpliciter tepefactum pluries *opturato* (obturato) ore et *foramina* (foraminibus) narium cum manu infirmi sufflando infirmus de sub osse expellebat saniem. *Nam* (et) saepe accessit quod labia vulneris ex abundantia carnis *crevit* (creverunt), sed tangendo cum tali aqua carnem illam dimenuebam, cuius descriptio talis est. Rx: salis gemmae, *alumen* (aluminis) rochiae, *vitrioli* (salis) armoniaci ana fiat distillitio *per* (ad) alembicum, *sed ista aqua* (et istam aquam) *operatur* (operantur) ab *aurificibus* (artifices), quando volunt *separare* (segregare) aurum ab argento. Sed antequam operarem ipsam (aquam) in vulnere ponebam spongiam vel bombicem, ne aqua *illa* (ista) *tangerit* (tangeret) quod non erat tangendum, et sic faciebam totiens quotiens erat opportunum.

Item aliquando ponebam ruptorium emum de alumine catino, *cuius* (quod) non posset clare scribi, nec lingua proferi; nisi videretur modus artificii *in componendo* et tantae proprietatis quod nullum *inferebat* nocumentum (infert) egrotanti. Sed habuisti aluid ruptorium supra quod dicitur capitellum, quod solum in tangendo carnem discoopertam a pelle *fit* (sit) satis notabile *diminutio*; cuius descriptio talis est.

Rx: primam aquam quam colligunt a vase illi qui volunt fa(e)cre saponem nigrum. Et ista talis aqua dicitur in vulgari sermone la magistra, que hoc modo fit. Sit unum vas amplum in fundo et strictum in superiori parte, ore [73r] reaperto plenum per partem post partem cineribus et *calcis* (calce) non extincta et cum aqua calida superius infusa; fac sicut lixivium per parvum foramen fundi inferius descendat. *Nec talis* (Hanc talem) aqua[m] collige vel

by various authors so I will be silent, for there is no need to describe it.

I do not apply anything stringent[58] to the opening unless, of course, it be simply warmed rose oil. Frequently, if the patient exhales, closing his mouth and his nares with his hand, he expels the discharge from under the bone. It often happens, moreover, that the lips of the wound heap up because of an abundance of flesh. This can be reduced by touching them with this liquid, the description of which is as follows. Rx: Rock salt, crude alum, ammoniac salt in equal parts. Distill in an alembic. This liquid is used by goldsmiths in separating gold from silver. Before applying this water, I insert a sponge[59] or piece of cotton[60] to prevent the liquid from reaching the undesired areas. I do this as often as is necessary.

Item. Sometimes I use my remover[61] of alum catino, which cannot be clearly described, neither by written word nor by tongue, unless you see it made, and it is of such property as to never harm the patient in any way. I have another remover which is called "a little head", since it is applied only to desquamated flesh. Its merit is singular, and its description is as follows:

Rx: The first water collected in the vase used to make black soap; this water is called in the vernacular "la magistra". It can also be made in the following fashion. Take a vase, wide at the bottom with a constriction in the upper part, and an open mouth. [73ʳ] Insert into it layers of ashes and hot lime. Fill to the top with warm water, permitting the lye[62] to descend through the small opening to the bottom. Collect this liquid, either according to the above instruction, or in the manner of those who make black soap. When you obtain this liquid, heat it gently until it boils, then remove it from the fire and save this ruptorium in jars. But take care lest you labor foolishly in this procedure. With this ruptorium I remove all the removable flesh, thus enlarging[63] the wound without either an incision, hemorrhage, or pain. I keep the wound open until the thirty-second day, at which time, or thereabouts, the physician attempts to remove the bone of the skull with the *moicula*. After this

---

[58]abstersivum
[59]spongiam
[60]bombicum
[61]ruptorium
[62]lixivum
[63]amplio

ex hoc magisterio supra habiro, ex doctrina data; vel ab hiis qui saponem nigrum *construiunt* (construunt). Sed habita ista talis aqua tamdiu cum suavi *ygne bullias* (igne buliat donec fiat sicut scis) *quod per ingrassationem fiat sicut lapis cocta habita super fernim vel lapidem* ab igne removeas et in ampulla hoc ruptorium serva. Sed *quando quomodo et qualiter operari oporteat non* (cavequomodo opereris ne) tamquam stultus *inane* (male) labores. Sed cum hoc ruptorio removebam *tantam* (totam) carnem quantum volebam *removere* et sic ampliabam vulnus sine incisione et fluxu sanguinis; et sine dolore ipsum vulnus tenendo apertum usque ad trigenta secundam diem, in qua die vel parem circa semper ossa a craneo, et tentata a medico si sunt removenda cum *molicula* (moicula) leviter *extrahitur* (extrahuntur); hoc facto et habito debes semper sequi naturam (ducem) in vulnus consolidando atque *rosbot* (arosboth) confirmando cum *cibariis* (cibis) viscosis, et absolutae *aprobatis* (appropriatis) sicut *furmentum* (frumentum) *cottum* (coctum), pisces *ciberia* (cibi) qui fiunt de pasta, caseus non salitus, et extremitates animalium ut sunt nervi *viscera* (viscere) *cotta* (cocta) et pedes *iuvencarum* (iuvencorum) et *pecudum* (aliorum animalium). Sed hoc facto, *scilicet*, osse remoto procedebam cum *isto* (hoc) tali unguento, quod pro (re)generanda pelle in capite, et pro cicatrizando multum valet, cuius descriptio talis est. Rx: minii olei rosati, de ambobus quantum est necesse. *Bulliantur in captio* (buliat in cacia) donec fiat ad formam unguenti, (et) sicut cerotum *et* extensibile super petiam cum *digito grosso* (digitis).

Item sicut dixi de minio *ita* posset fieri simili modo, *unguentum* de litargiro unguentum, aut de cerusa cum oleo rosato ad formam duram et simili modo extensibilia, quae unguenta sunt aliquando generative carnis, que generative carnis non est aluid *nisi* (quam) coagulatio sanguinis in carnem. Et *haec* (loco) talis operatio completur per primum gradum siccitatis, et parum plus respectu membri, cui tale medicamem (operatur et) *aplicabatur* (applicatur). Alquando haec medicina est incarnativa quae incarnatio fit per secundum gradum siccitatis, et haec talis incarnatio perficitur quando duo labia elongata ad invicem conglutinatur.

Item haec unguenta cicatrizativa. Nam cicatrizare, ut supra dictum est in capitulo de medicinis cicatrizantibus *nichil* (nihil) aliud est, nisi carnem aliqualiter indurare. Et haec talis operatio completur per tertium gradum siccitatis *carnem* indurando, taliter quod humidum substantificum nullum inferat nocumentum in parte ex-

has been done, following the tendency of nature to condense[64] the wound, you always ought to strengthen the callus[65] with viscid food and such indispensible necessities as cooked grain, fish, pasta, unsalted cheese, the extremities of animals, such as legs of cows and other animals, as well as cooked nerves and viscera. This done, i.e., when the bone is removed, I proceed with this ointment. It is useful in regenerating[66] the skin of the scalp and in promoting a scar. Its description is: red lead, oil of roses, ambobaja of sufficient quantity. Boil in an urn until it has the consistency of an ointment. Spread above the part with the fingers.

Item. What I have stated concerning cinnabar can, in the same fashion, be said about litharge or ceruse with rose oil in the hard form. They are applied in similar fashion since all these ointments promote granulation.[67] Granulation is nothing more than the congealment of blood into flesh. This process is completed through the first stage of desiccation,[68] more or less depending on that structure to which these medicines are applied. Sometimes this medicine promotes healing,[69] for healing is the second stage of desiccation and comes about when the elongated two lips approach one another and stick together.

Item. These are cicatrizing[70] ointments, for, as said in the Capitulum *De Medicina Cicatrizantibus*, scar tissue differs in no way from flesh except in the way in which it hardens. This process[71] is completed through three stages of desiccation. If the flesh becomes hard in such a way that the substantive moisture[72] does no harm to the exterior of the part by corrupting itself in the scar, then this scar will be handsome. After finishing with the plaster, I next apply an ointment over the defect in the patient's head. Over this I place a small cupping glass, which is perforated in many places. There are three reasons for using this cupping glass. First, lest the drains compress by pressure from the dressing or the pillows. Second, so that the discharge can escape from the wound even though the

---

[64]consolido
[65]arosboth
[66]regenerando
[67]gerativa carnis
[68]siccitatis
[69]incarnativa
[70]cicatrizativa
[71]operatio
[72]humidum substantificum

teriori se in *superficie* (cicatrice) corrumpendo, et hec talis cicatrix *est* (erit) puchra. Sed dimisso emplastro huic infirmo supra foramen cranei prius posito unguento *aposui unum petium* (apposui unam petium) cucurbitae (id est zuche) in pluribus locis perforatae. Et haec aposito cucurbitae potest poni *propter* (per) tres causas; prima *causa ut* ne stuelii in vulneribus propter aliquam compressionem quae fieri posset a ligatura aut a pulvinaribus su[b]mergantur et lesionem faciant. Secunda causa ne per compressionem ligamentorum sanies extra vulnus possit expelli fiunt foramina ut sanies usque ad superficiem tam intrinsecam quam extrinsecam possit *transpirare* (respirare). Tertia causa cucurbita *aponitur* (ponitur) in magnis fracturis capitis; quia est corpus leve et sine aliqua mala complexione, et prohibet ne aer extrinsecus cerebrum alteret. Et hoc *petium* (frustum) cucurbitae debet [ap]poni et sine foraminibus quando non *a*ponitur emplastrum capitale, quod fieri non potest causa necessitatis, et quando est magnum frigus.

Hoc (Haec) autem de cucurbita tangere volui propter *removere* (removendam) errone[a]m *et* opinonem ydiotarum *dicendo* (dicentium) partes cucurbitarum *sunt* (esse) in capitibus aliquorum. Sed *quod* hoc *sit* (esse) incredibile sic demonstratur per istam rationem. Nam si cucurbita incarnaretur, tunc *non bene et secure operetur a medico et a natura quae semper agit pro sua conservatione* (medicus qui laborat propter conservationem natura non recte operaretur). Nam cum ossa sint magis dura, et sibi ipsi craneo magis consimilia deberent etiam incarnari, et ut visum est per experientiam *et per raciocinationem* [73v] non incarnantur, dum illud os sit totaliter ablatum. Neque ergo cucurbita quae est alterius speci ab osse humani capitis. *Sic ergo* (itaque) stultum est et erroneum credere.

In trigentaquarto die *supervenit isto meo egritanti quinque* (habui unum ergo tantem, cui supervenit) *parosismos* (paroxismus) epilepsiae, sive *quinque parosismos* (paroxismus) spasmi, quod idem (est), cum communis epilepsia sit spasmus *sed* (et) non e converso. Sed quia *fui* (aderam) presens in quatro *parosixmo* (paroxismo) prohibui inquantum potui cum diversivis, scilicet, ligando extrema cum *victis* (alutis) et erigendo ipsum subiectum rectum et elevatum cum capite, et in auribus ponendo casturnum, quod est in hoc casu *de meis secretis et* de mirabilibus mundi, et *similiter quod valoret citius* (citius valet) sub lingua *idem iuvamentum*.

Item (in) collo (ipsius) infirmi *suspensi* (suspendi) in sacculo radicem peoniae pulverizatam.

dressings cover it. Holes are made so that the intrinsic as well as extrinsic discharge can evaporate anywhere on the surface. Third, cups are placed in large skull fractures since they are light, harmless, and a protection to the cerebrum from injury by the outside air. This small cup should not contain holes, however, when there is no need for a plaster to be placed on the head nor should it have holes when it is very cold.

In the following I wish to touch upon cups in order to refute the mistaken opinions of foolish men who say that there are parts of cupping glass in some people's heads! That these fallacies are incredible is demonstrated by this reasoning: if the cup turn into flesh, then the doctor who labors for the conservation of nature labors improperly. Since bones are very hard and very similar to the cranium itself, they too ought to turn into flesh, but as seen through experience *and through reasoning*, [73^{v}] they do not become flesh if that bone is completely removed. Therefore, the cup which is of another substance than the human head, does not either, for this is quite silly and he who believes it is in error.

In the thirty-fourth day one very sick patient experienced epileptic seizures or spastic paroxysms which are the same since spasm accompanies epilepsy and not the converse. During these episodes I was present. I was able to stop the fourth seizure by diverse means, e.g., by binding the extremity with leather,[73] stretching out the patient so that he was straight, elevating his head, and by placing castor in his ear, which, in this situation, worked wonders, but acted more quickly when placed under the tongue.

Item. Around the neck of the patient I suspend a sack of powdered root of peonie.

Item. Always have the patient drink honey syrup, made from honey and water.

Item. I give him one measure of gladiola root electuary that same day, which has the ability to soothe nerves. This is its description: Rx: Gladiola root, rye of each 1 pound; fruit of pine 1 pound; black pepper 1 ounce; long peppers, cloves, ginger, galega of each half an ounce; Paradise grain, nutmeg, 3 drams; honey of sufficient quantity. Make an electuary. Wonderful in soothing nerves.

Item. In this sickness I commence digestion on the thirty-eighth day with this method. Rx: Syrup of lavender, syrup of mint

[73]alutis

Item semper mellicratum bibere feci, *quod* (et) fit ex aqua et melle.

Item electarium *de diacoro* (dedi) sibi (acori) unum cocleare in die semel *aposetavi*, quod habet virtutem mundificandi nervos, cuius descriptio *talis est* Rx: acori, rinci ana libra i; *pemarum* (pincarum) libra iss; piperis nigri unc. iss piperis longi gariofilorum, zinziber, galange ana unc. ss; cardamoni, nucis muscate ana dr. iii; mellis *quod* (quantum) sufficit, et fiat electuarium *et istud electuarium* est (quidem) divinum in mundificando nervos.

Item incepi digerere *materiam in iste ergo in 38ª die* (in hoc egro) hoc modo. Rx: syrupi de sticados, syrupi de menta ana unc. ss; aqua lauri (tauri), aqua mentae ana unc. ss; digesta materia evacuavi cum pilleris *ch*ochiis et aggregativis ana scrup. i; et faciebam quandoque fieri pilleras. His (autem) evacuationibus *vero* completis remansit vere debilitas in brachio, et in pede ex parte contraria vulneris, *et fracture* et hoc est propter cruciationem nervorum. Sed hoc modo removi illam, scilicet cum unctionibus et fumigiis. *Sed* (Et) unctiones fuerunt tales. Rx: olei de lateribus, olei de piperibus ana unc. ss; olei de terbentina, olei de costo ana dr. iii; oleo *volpini* (vulpini) dr. ii; fiat unguentum cum sufficienti cera alba. Suffumigia *fuerunt talia* (sunt haec). Rx: pumicem vel marchasitam si *habere* (haberi) *potes* (potest), sed ego *accepi lapidem* (accipiebam lapidis) molaris unum frustum *rubeum de quo acruentur ferramenta* et feci in igne accendi, et lapide ignito acetum fortissimum supra *prohicere* (proiicere) feci, et *femum cum pannis membrum bene copertum* (ad fumum membrum pannis bene coopertum) et o[b]turatum versus partem lesam, imponebat virtutem incisivam et revolutivam et ex*s*iccativam et confortativam in ipso membro qua propter membrum fortiter sudabat, et cum pannis ipsum tegebam, et cum unguento antedicto inungebam, et hoc feci bis in die donec eger sanus *ille* factus est, et incepit ambulare, et cum brachio suo *lesio et* paraliticato corporeum e[xe]git *exercitium* (officium).

V

Capitulum de ordinatione receptarum in fracturis et percussionibus a principio usque ad finem secundum tempora. Et primo de principio. Secundo de augmento. Tertio de statu. Quatro de declinatione, tractando de emplastris, et de unguentis, et de liquoribus, et de unctionibus, et de omnibus necessariis ut novus *cyroicus* (cyrurgicus) sciat modum applicandi.

of each half an ounce; laurel water *from the Bogni de Perrata*, mint water of each 1 ounce. After considerable digestion I evacuate with snail pills and hortense of each 1 scruple; and use the pellory whenever needed. After such a complete evacuation, the patient's arm and foot remain quite debilitated because of contraries in the wound, as a consequence of nerve pain.[74] This I remove by ointments and fumigation.[75] The ointments are as follows: Rx: Brick oil, oil of peppers of each half an ounce; oil of turpentine; cost oil of each 3 drams; fox oil 2 drams. Make an ointment with sufficient white wax. Fumigations[76] are these: Rx: Pumice or marchasitas, if available, but I might take one piece of millstone and, heating it into flames, sprinkle vinegar over the heated stone, exposing the lesion to the vapor. The extremity is well covered with dressings. Such dressings have the qualities of resolving and cleansing, and are most comforting. In this way the structure sweats profusely. I cover the wound with this dressing. With the aforementioned salve I anoint the wound, performing this twice daily until the patient recovers, begins to walk and moves his paralyzed limb.

Chapter V

Section concerning appropriate prescribing for fractures and concussions from early to final stages. First, concerning the early

[74]cruciatio
[75]fumigia
[76]suffumigia

Primum remedium *quod debet fieri* quando facta est solutio in capite, ad hoc ne materia fluat ad locum et ut sanguis retineatur. Rx: albumina ovorum *in* numero secundum necissitatem et bene conquassata, et pulveris boli armeni, et sanguinis draconis, et misce cum stuellis in vulnere positis et madefactis *in* (cum) hoc liquore, et cum faldelis stupeis *similiter* (prius) madefactis primitus in aqua frigida, (aut vino nigro) et ab *aqua* (eo) expressis si times, vel sit fluxus sanguinis; si vero non times *et non* (nec) sit fluxus sanguinis madefac prius *ipsas* (dictas) faldelas in vino nigro et postea in albuminibus ovorum bene conquassatorum et appone supra locum vulneratum, et supra stuellos et liga cum fascia debito modo *et sic* (sicque) procede ad duas vel (ad) tres mutationes cum dicto remedio [74r]

Aliud remedium sequens ad istud in principio, quod communiter solet fieri causa sedandi dolorem, et causa digerendi materiam coniunctam in vulnere. Rx: unum vitellum ovi recentem, et *apone intus* (impone interius) de oleo rosato recenti et non antiquo, et *in*simul misce, et stuellis in hoc unguento madefactis vulnere a[p]pone usque ad tres vel ad *quator* (quatro) mutationes, *vel* donec vulnus incipiat saniari. Sed circumcirca vulnus oleum rosatum *calidum* semper ponatur, ut (dolor) mitigetur, et ut repercutiat humores de novo venientes ad locum, et ut confortet partes membri circumstantes, (et) propter stipticitatem olei rosati quam habet ratione rosarum.

Item (valet etiam) oleum rosatum et potest poni supra stuellos eos humectando donec in *vulnus* (vulnere) fiat digestio.

Item. Emplastrum quod debet poni in fractura capitis *et hoc* in augmento. Rx: maioranae, betonice, assari, foliorum lauri, calamenti, florum camomille et melliloti et matri silvae ana M. i; farinae ordei M. ii; et olei rosati unc. iiii; et cum aqua decoctionis ordei fiat emplastrum.

Unguentum quod debet poni in vulnere (in augmento) et in statu, ut materia digeratur, et saniata abstergatur (et valet etiam in statu). Rx: olei rosati *de* recenti[s] et non de antiquo unc. ss; mellis rosati collati dr. ii; omnia insimul misce, et tepefactur stuellos in *hoc* liquore madefactor *vulneri* (vulnere) a[p]pone.

Unguentum quod supra stuellos et vulnus debet a[p]poni est tale. Rx: resinae pini bene (tersae et) mundae unc. ii; olei rosati unc. i; cere quod sufficit. Fiat unguentum et adde in fine pulveris sandaracae, pulveris gummi elemi ana dr. i.

stage; second, the stage of augmentation; third, the establishment;[77] fourth, the decline.[78] In this section I describe plasters, ointment, liquids, ointments and all the things the young surgeon should know about their application.

The first remedy for an open head wound is used, lest material flow to the site and blood be retained. Rx: A sufficient quantity of whipped egg white, powdered Armenian pills and dragon blood. Soak these in the drain and place the drain in the wound. If you anticipate bleeding or if it has already started, soak a wool stupe in cold water and squeeze out the excess. If you do not fear the outcome and blood is not present, wet the aforesaid wool first in black wine and afterwards in whipped egg white. Then place it over the wound site and above the drain, fastening the drain as required with a bandage.[79] Proceed in this way [74^r] through two to three changes with the above.

Another remedy used after the foregoing in the beginning of the illness, with which one frequently can soothe pain and digest material retained[80] in the wound. Rx: One fresh egg yolk. Add to it fresh—not stale—rose oil, mix, moisten a drain in this ointment and place it into the wound. Apply the drain through three or four changes in the wound until the wound begins to look healthy. Around the wound anoint rose oil to soothe the pain, to repress[81] the humors flowing to the site and to comfort the structures surrounding the lesion. It does this by the styptic action of rose oil which it owes to the presence of the roses.

Item. Rose oil is useful. It can be placed over the drain. Moisten it until digestion begins in the wound.

Item. A plaster which should be used for the fractured skull in the stage of augmentation. Rx: Majory, betony, asarabacca, laurel leaves, calaminth, flowers of camomile, meliot, honeysuckle of each 1 fistful; barley meal 2 fistsful; oil of roses 4 ounces; and barley water. Make a plaster.

An ointment used in the stage of augmentation and in the stage of establishment to digest material and cleanse the discharge. Rx: Fresh oil of roses half an ounce; red honey cooked 2 drams.

---

[77]status
[78]declinatio
[79]fascia
[80]conjuncta
[81]repercute

Unguentum aliud capitale quod valet ad fracturam cranei et est optimum. Rx: millefolii, berbenae, bettonicae centauree, maiorane ana M. ss; omnes istae herbae diligenter laventur *que* (et) postea in mortario diligenter pistentur, et cum vino maluatico incorporentur et per tres vel quatuor dies (cum predicto) vino in mortario *permictantur* (dimmittantur) postea ad ygnem (ignem) cum *captia* (cacia) nitida buliantur, et semper cum spatula *lignea* misceantur *insimul* donec virtus herbarum incorporetur, (et) postea coletur. Hoc facto Rx: cere *virginis* (citrinae) lib. ss et dr. ii; terbentine *bone* (bene) (lotae cum vino albo) et *clare* (claro) lib. ss et incorporentur omnia ista *cum predicto* (in dicto) vino colato, et tamdiu *bulliantur* (buliant) insimul quod dici possim *septiem* (septies) pater noster et semper lento *ygne de* coquatur, et semper cum spatula lignea *permiseatur* (agitetur), et postea deponatur ab ygne igne), et *dimictatur* (dimittatur) infrigidari et coagulari, et quando coagulatum fuerit ponatur *pulveris* (pulvis) aristologiae rotundea unc. ss; olei rosati coclearia x; et incorporentur cum *predicto* (dicto) unguento et *dimictatur* (dimmittatur) stare sic *consectus per tres vel quator* (per duos aut tres) dies in succo be*t*tonicae et aliarum herbarum supradictarum et semper istis diebus miscendo postea in fine *istarum* (istorum) dierum coletur per petiam subtilem et nitidam, et usui reserva, et valet ad vulnera capitis cum petia incisa et *folia* (folio) cavlis et etiam valet ad alia vulnera.

Unguentum aliud in fractura cranei miabile et bonum. Rx: cere albe unc. i; terbentine dr. ii; ista duo bul*l*iant in succo istarum herbarum (scilicet) be*t*tonicae et *mille folii* (milefolii) centauree *maioris* (minoris) berbenae, postea extrahatur ab istis succis, et addantur *ista* (istae) cum istis, sciliet Rx: storacis calamenti unc. i; resine pini unc. ss; et incorporentur insimul et *prohisciantur* (proiiciantur) in aceto; postea de aceto extrahantur et *prohiciantur* (proiiciantur) in lacte mulieris, et cum manibus bene ducatur et usui *postea* reservetur.

Unguentum aliud de *rasina* (resina) quod est valde attractivum et optimum bonum. Rx: olei communis unc. iii; cere unc. i; rasinae pini dr. ss; Galbani in aceto dissoluti unc. ss; terbentinae clarae dr. ii; croci scrup. i; et fiat unguentum. [74^{v}]

Unguentum aliud (valde) bonum. Rx: pimpinelle, berbenae be*t*tonica[e] ana M. i; herbe iste omnes laventur et pistentur et *permictantur* (dimittantur) stare quinque (v) diebus cum una quarta parte boni vini albi, postea bul*l*iantur et colentur et in colatura predicta ponantur omnia ista. Scilicet Rx: cere Virginis unc. ii;

Mix together and moisten the drain in warm liquid. Place it over the wound.

An ointment which should be placed above the drain and the wound. Rx: Purifed and first quality resin of pine 2 ounces; oil of roses 1 ounce; wax of sufficient quantity. Make an ointment and add powdered sandara, powdered gummi elemi of each 1 dram.

Another very valuable ointment for fractured skulls: Rx: Marrow, pimpernelle, betony, century major of each half a fistful. Wash these herbs well and grind thoroughly in a mortar, incorporating with Malvasia wine. Allow the mixture to stand for 3 to 4 days in the mortar with the wine. Afterwards, heat with good quality senna and mix with a spatula until the herbs are incorporated. Then strain. Rx: Yellow wax half a pound and 2 drams; turpentine well-washed with clear white wine half a pound; incorporate all in the wine after it has been strained. Thereafter, boil everything for the length of time it takes to say seven Pater Nosters. Then stir over a gentle fire with the wooden spatula and afterwards take out of the fire and allow to cool and coagulate, adding thereafter powdered aristolochia round half an ounce; oil of roses 10 tablespoons. Incorporate with the said ointment and allow to stand for two or three days in betony, sugar and the above herbs. At the end of this time wash and strain through a thin sieve. Save for later use. It is of value for head wounds and even for other wounds as well.

Another wonderful and useful ointment for fractured skulls. Rx: White wax 1 ounce; turpentine 2 drams; boil these in the juice of such herbs as betony, milfoil, lesser century, pimpernel. Afterwards remove from these juices and add: Rx: Storax, calaminth 1 ounce; resin of pine half an ounce. Incorporate and sprinkle in mother's milk. Knead well with your hands and save for later use.

Another excellent ointment. Rx: Pimpernel, betony of each 1 fistful. Those praiseworthy herbs are washed, ground and allowed to stand for five days in one quadroon of good white wine. Then they are boiled and strained. Into the material to be strained the following are placed: Rx: Green wax 2 ounces. At the end of the cooking process add 1 ounce of good wine and permit the mixture to boil in the wine to form a hard substance from which pastilles are made. Always mix over a gentle fire and allow to stand.

Another excellent resin ointment which is good and is a powerful attractor.[82] Rx: Common oil 3 ounces; wax 1 ounce; resin of

[82]attractivum

postea in fine decoctionis addatur unc. iss optimi vini, et tamen permittatur bul/ire cum predicto vino quod veniat in substantia dura ut possi[n]t inde fieri magdaliones et semper miscendo igne lento, et postea recondatur.

Unguentum aliud *et perfectum* in fractura cranei. Rx: succi salviae, succi maiorane, succi matri[s] silvae, succi serpilii ana dr. ss; olei rosati et cere quantum sufficit, et fiat unguentum cui addatur in fine decoctionis pulveris bdelii, pulveris gummi elemi, pulveris serapini, pulveris foliorum folii ana dr. ss. Fiat unguentum.

Unguentum in fractura cranei quod usus fui et habui honorem. Rx: rasinae pini, albe et electae unc. ii; olei rosati unc. i; cere albae dr. iii; omnia dissolvantur insimul per optime ad *ygnem* (ignem) et colentur et infundantur in vino albo, et adde in fine *modicum* (parum) de minio et operetur, postea extendendo *istud* (illud) unguentum supra petiam.

Experimentum *consiliatoris* (conciliatoris) seu magistri *(petri* (luce) de abano quod curat fracturas cranei absque elevatione ossis, unde lege *consilietorem* (conciliatorem) quia dicit hoc experimentum (in) doctrinia *181*[a]. (Idem illa.) Rx: gummi elemi unc. iii; *rasine* (resinae) pini purissime unc. iiii cere unc. iiii; olei rosati *unc. iii* (unc. ii); armoniaci unc. ii; terbentinae unc. iii et dr. v. Fiat unguentum, et quidam addunt in eo farinam siliginis quidam conponunt cum vino absque oleo et cera, et *possit* (posset) fieri post principium.

Unguentum valde *optimum* (bonum) in fractura cranei. Rx: gummi elemi dr. iii; oppoponacis dr. ii; bdellii dr. iss; *rasine* (resinae) pini unc. i; cere alba quantum sufficit. Fiat unguentum.

Aliud unguentum *solepne* (solemne) in fractura cranei. Rx: gummi ceresorum, gummi persicorum, gummi elemi ana unc. iii; resinae pini albae et bene pulchrae unc. iiii; *populari sive minii vel* (seu) cere citrinae unc. v; olei rosati unc. iiii; armoniaci unc. ii; terbentinae unc. iii. Fiat unguentum et malaxetur cum bono vino montano odorifero.

Emplastrum conveniens cum unguentis ana scriptis. Rx: calamenti, sticados arabici, foliorum lauri et salviae et roris marini ana M. i; camomille, melliloti, *asari* (assari) ana unc. i; croci scrup. i; olei liliorum alborum, olei *camomillin* (camomellini) ana unc. i. Fiat emplastrum cum decoctione ordei, et istud emplastrum debet [ap]poni quando *in capite* vulnus esset cum contusione.

Emplastrum valde mirabile ad elevandum os cranei depressum quod saepe contigit in pueris quando cadunt *vel oviant* (et obviant

pine half a dram; galbanum dissolved in vinegar half an ounce; clear turpentine 2 drams; saffron 1 scruple. Make an ointment. [74^{v}]

Another ointment. Rx: Syrup of sage, syrup of majory, syrup of honeysuckle, syrup of wild thyme of each half a dram; oil of roses and wax of sufficient quantity. Make an ointment to which is added, after it is cooked, powdered bdellium, powdered gum elemi, powdered serapinum, powdered beans of each half a dram. Make an ointment.

Another ointment which I favor and respect for fractured skulls. Rx: Resin of choice white pine 2 ounces; oil of roses 1 ounce; white wax 3 drams. Dissolve well by heating, strain and collect in white wine, adding a little quantity of red lead, then cover. Afterwards apply this ointment over the part.

An experiment from the Conciliator, or Master Peter of Abano, which cures fractures without the need for elevating the bone. You may consult the Conciliator, for he describes this experiment in his 181st doctrine. Rx: Gum elemi 3 ounces; resin of pine, very pure wax 4 ounces; oil of roses 2 ounces; armoniac 2 ounces; turpentine 3 ounces and 5 drams. Make an ointment.

Another fine ointment for fractured skulls. Rx: Gum elemi 3 drams; opoponax 2 drams; bdellium 1 dram; resin of pine 1 ounce; white wax of sufficient quantity. Make an ointment.

Another venerable ointment for treating fractured skulls. Rx: Gum of white wax, gum of heart wort, resin of myrrh of each 3 ounces; resin of attractive white pine 4 ounces; storax or yellow wax 5 ounces; oil of roses 4 ounces; armoniac 2 ounces; turpentine 3 ounces. Make an ointment and add good mountain wine with a fragrant bouquet.

An appropriate plaster with an ointment of the following description. Rx: Calaminth, lavender, laurel leaves, sage, rosemary of each 1 fistful; camomile, meliot, asarabacca of each 1 ounce; saffron 1 scruple; oil of white lilies, oil of camomile of each 1 ounce. Make a plaster with cooked barley and place above a contused wound.

An excellent plaster for elevating depressed bones, such as often occurs when children fall and strike a hard object. Rx: Ordinary honey 1 pound; cook over a fire and add fermented bran 1 pound; sulfur 2 drams; common salt 2 ounces; cinnamon, wormwood of each 2 drams. Make a plaster.

rei durae) *aliquam rem duram*. Rx: mellis communis lib. iss; coquatur ad ignem et addantur ista, scilicet furfuris f[r]umenti lib. i; sulfuris dr. ii; salis communis unc. ii; cimini, absinthii ana dr. ii. Fiat emplastrum.

Istud enim emplastrum multotiens expertus fui, et vidi ossa capitis depressa in pueris mirabiliter elevare in quindecim diebus.

Emplastrum mirabile, et est unum experimentum ad cognoscendum utrum craneum sit fractum vel non, nulla lesione apparens exterius et est a multis expertum. Rx: thuris cere, laudani ana unc. iii pulverizentur et incorporentur ad invicem, et fiat emplastrum, capite prius abrase *superponitur* (superponatur) et per noctem unam *dimictatur* (dimittatur) in mane *vero* (autem) removeatur, *sed* (et) ubi lesio fuerit pars ipsius cutis [75r] erit desiccata, et per istud experimentum potes cognoscere lesionem si fuerit in osse.

Emplastrum aliud secundum quod audivi a *valentissimis medicis et* (prudentissimis) doctoribus quod (fit) certificatio de fractura cranei quando dubitatur, et non apparet lesio per hoc experimentum potest sciri. Rx: cere, laudani, thuris ana lib. i; terbentinae, farinae, fabarum, aceti ana lib. ss; dissolvantur omnia, et bene malazentur, ut sint extensibilia, deinde fiat ex eis ad modum bereti (bireti), et super capite extendatur per noctem, capillis abrasis prius mane vero suaviter [e]llevetur et *invenietur* (invenies) biretum ibi in parte cranei lesi quodammodo perforatum, aut diminutum aliquantulum

Emplastrum aliud ad reducendum plicatum os ad *anteriora* (interiora) quod *plerumque* (quandoque) accidit in *capite* (capitibus) puerorum. Rx: mel apum, et lapidem magnetis et salem et pumicem et pulverizanda pulverizentur, et insimul omnia misceantur, et fiat emplastrum et usui reserva.

Emplastrum de matri silve optimum in capite fracto, et si vis potes facere *ad* (in) formam unguenti. Rx: foliorum matri(s) silvae, et fiat suc[c]us, olei communis ana lib. ss; cere unc. iiii; terbentinae, *rasine* (resinae) pini ana unc. iii; bul*l*iantur omnia usque ad consumptionem succi, et fiat emplastrum vel unguentum secundum quod vis.

Emplastrum optimum capitale. Rx: fluorum camomelle, *et* mel[l]iloti calamenti, origani, sticados arabici ana unc. ss; olei *camomillini* (camomelline) anetini ana unc. ii; *butiri* (butyri) sine sale unc. iss; mellis unc. iii; farinae ordei quod sufficit, et fiat emplastrum.

With this ointment I was often able to treat effectively and have seen a depressed skull fracture in children wondrously elevated in fifteen days.

A wondrous plaster which is also an experiment for determining whether or not the skull is fractured, when there is no lesion apparent on the surface. Rx: Olibanum, wax, laudanum of each 3 ounces; pulverize and incorporate, making a plaster, and apply it above the shaved head. Leave it for one night. In the morning remove it and where a lesion is present part of the skin [75^r] will be dried up. By means of this experiment you will be able to know if a bone lesion is present.

Another plaster learned from prudent physicians, who used it to establish the diagnosis of skull fracture in doubtful cases where a lesion was absent. Rx: Wax, laudanum, olibanum of each 1 pound; turpentine, bean meal, vinegar of each half a pound. Dissolve all and mix well so that it is stretchable, and apply over the head for one night, fashioning a little cap. But first cut the hair. In the morning lift up gently and you will find the cap in that part of the skull where it is perforated or thinned out to any extent.

Another plaster for elevating [depressed fractures], such as occur in young children. Rx: Honey, magnetic rock, salt and pumice. Grind all to a powder and mix simultaneously. Make a plaster. Save it for future use.

An excellent plaster of honeysuckle for fractured skulls which can be made up in ointment form. Rx: Leaves of honeysuckle and make a syrup, common oil of each half a pound; wax 4 ounces; turpentine, resin of each 3 ounces. Boil all until the syrup dissolves. Make a plaster or ointment as desired.

An excellent plaster. Rx: Flowers of camomile, meliot, calaminth, pennyroyal, lavender, gum arabic of each half a dram; oil of camomile, dill of each 2 drams; saltless butter 3 drams; barley meal of sufficient quantity. Make a plaster.

A plaster compounded by *Gentile* from resin of myrrh which is a soothing salve to the discharge and to the structures under the bone, wondrously elevating bone fragments. Rx: Armoniac, bdellium, serapinum, galbanum, oponopnax, resin of myrrh of each half an ounce; turpentine, naval pitch, resin of pine, oak sap, leftovers of a dish of anchovies of each 3 ounces; aristolochia round and long, dittany, colphony, myrrh, an ox stone, polypody, bark of aruninacea root of each 3 drams; leaven, pig's fat, laurel oil of each

Unguentum compositum a *Gentile* (Gentili) de gummi elemi, et est unguentum mundificativum saniei, *de* (et) sub osse, et frustrum ossis elevans mirabiliter. Rx: armoniaci, bdellii, serapini, galbani, oppoponaci[s], gummi elemi ana unc. ss; terbentine, picis navalis, rasinae pini, visci quercini *sorditiei* (sordiciei) vasorum *apum* (apium) ana unc. iii; aristologiae rotunde et *lon* (longe), diptami, colofoniae, mirrae lapidis, calamite pol[l]ipodii, *corticum* (cortices) radicis arundinis ana dr. iii; fermenti, *asungie* (axungiae) porcinae, olei laurini ana unc. ii aceti unc. ii. Fiat unguentum cum sufficienti cera et additione (sordiciei) *vasorum* (vasum) apum supradicte, vel mellis loco eius, et olei *aneti sufficietur* (anetini quod sufficit).

Unguentum ad formam liquoris quod extrahit abstergit saniem de sub osse, et de ubicumque locorum. Rx: succi betonicae et mellis rosati colati ana unc. i; et misce insimul et decoquatur usque ad consumptionem succi, et postea adde gummi pulversis elemi et *prohiciatur* (proiiciatur) in vulnere et fac quod eger sufflet *saniem* (sanies) *ad extra obturatis naribus et ore* (nares obturando, et os) cum manu.

Dieta istorum vulneratorum in capite fuit, non sint cum vulnere sed cum fractura a principio usque ad decem dies si fuerit in estate. In hyeme usque ad septimam diem donec fueris securus ab apostemate. (Dieta istorum vulneratorum in capite, sive sint cum vulnere sive absque fractura debet esse a principio usque ad decem dies si fuerit in aestate, usque ad septimum, si autem in hyeme debes expectare usque ad decem dies, sed si contusio fuerit magna, ut verbi gratia quod ceciderit de alto debes expectare usque ad xvi diem, quamvis nihil accidit in octavo, et hic est cibus quo potest uti.) Rx: micam panis (albissimi) lotam in aqua, et bulita[m] in ipsa aqua sine sale *et cum uno vitello ovi prius posito* (sal namque est durae digestionis, deinde addatur unum vitellum ovi prius positum) ad macerandum in aqua frigida, *et istud erit unum ministrum quod paduani vocant panatam id est* (erit conveniens cibus, et vocatur communiter panata), cibus factus ex pane et aqua *decoctis*. Item addere potes succum farri[s] aut suc[c]us ordei, lactucas, boragines conditas cum lacte *amigdolarum* (amigdalarum) et cucurbitas cum eodem lacte, et hoc fiat, si virtus fuerit fortis. Sed si virtus fuerit debilis des ei carnes edi (edorum) pullorum (minutorum) coctas cum cucurbita lactuca *portulace* (portulaca) cum agresta vel cum vino de pomis *granatorium* (granatis) et utatur ista dieta donec fueris securus ab apostemate calido, et donec craneum sit *perfectum* (perfecte) incarnatum cum dura matre. Postea da infirmo de *capietti arietis* (capitibus, aut) pedibus [75v] vitulorum (aut capiti) de caseo non

2 ounces; vinegar 1 ounce. Make an ointment with sufficient wax and add bee waste as mentioned above or honey in lieu and dill oil of sufficient quantity.

An ointment in the form of a liquid which removes and cleanses[83] the discharge from under the bone, or wherever it is located. Rx: Sugar of betony and red honey strained of each 1 ounce. Mix and cook together until the syrup is dissolved, adding thereafter powdered resin of myrrh. Apply to the wound and have the patient exhale the discharge through his nose, squeezing his nostrils and covering his mouth with his hands.

In those patients having head wounds with or without fractures, this is the diet to be used from the beginning to the tenth day in winter or the seventh day in summer; or, to the sixteenth day if the contusion be great, such as happens, for example, when the fall was from a great height, even though nothing untoward occurs on the eighth. Rx: White bread crumbs bathed in water and boiled without salt, salt being difficult to digest. Then I add an egg yolk beat up in cold water, which is a good food and is commonly called pancake, a food made of bread and water. I then add wheat meal or barley meal, lettuce, heliotrope with milk of almonds and melon juice, administering this if the patient's strength be strong. If his strength be weak,give him pullet meat cooked with melon, lettuce, wild purslain or with pomegranate wine. Keep him on this diet until he is safe from the danger of hot pus and until the skull as well as the dura mater is perfectly healed.[84] After, give the patient the head or feet [75^{v}] of veal, or unsalted cheese and cooked grain so that gross and viscid humors are generated, these being necessary that they be transformed into hard and callous substances to replace the removed bone. Moreover, for dessert the patient may eat stewed apples and pears, capons and small nestling birds, as long as they do not come from the swamp. Until the end of the cure always caution the patient to refrain from wine.

Wine draws much material from the head to the brain, *and causes debilitation to the brain and passage of the humors to the head*. Therefore, the patient is to be content with water boiled with kernels of wild bread or fermented grain mixed with water or barley meal cooked with old red sugar. All this comforts the mouth of the stomach and since the stomach is connected to the cerebrum through sympathy by means of nerves from the brain to the mouth

[83]abstergo
[84]incarnatum

salito de *langanis de* frumento cocto *in ministro* ut generetur grossus humor et viscosus, ad hoc ut sit conveniens *ad conversionem* (converti) in rem duram et calosam loco ossis deperditi, et comedat poma et pira cocta sub prunis post cibum, et cum hoc potest comedere pullos gallinas, aves minutas *de nidis in arborius et non in vallibus* (quae sint adhuc in nido, dummodo non sint ortae in paludinibus). Et (semper) custodiatur infirmus usque ad perfectam curationem a vino.

Vinum enim multum trahit materias in capite ad cerebrum *et inducit debilitatem cerebri et cursum humorum ad cerebrum*. Sit ergo contentus *in* aqua *decoctionem medulle* (decocta communi medulla) panis agresta vel vino granatorum cum aqua mixto vel aqua ordei cocta excorticata, et cum zucharo rosato veteri, omnia ista confortant os stomaci, et propter affinitatem quam habet cum cerebro ex nervo current a cerebro ad os stomaci, et propter hanc affinitatem ex compassione currunt humores ad os stomaci, *et ad stomacum expercussione sit vomitus et hic tales dicta comfortat stomacum* et *inpedit* (inpediunt) fumos ascendentes ad caput. Si autem infirmus vellet pur bibere vinum, (bibat), *capiat* vinum, aquosum debile et bruscum de plano, et cum aqua cocta parum zuc[h]arata, et sic vinum ponticum, et aqua in duplici quantitate ipsius vini.

Dieta vero illius qui non habet fracturam in craneo, *ymo* (immo) solum vulnus in *cute* (cuti) et in panniculo almocati teneat dietamusque ad *otto* (octo) dies, donec medicus sit securus de apostemate calido, postea revertatur ad consolidationem *suam* debitam et convenientem (ponendo istud capitulum ad alia capitula). *Pone istud capitulum in aliis capitulis.*

Nota quod medici omnes practicantes hunc casum de fractura cranei et solutione capitis semper procedunt cum oleo rosato et cum mele rosato, et bene faciunt.

VI

Capitulum (Sequitur) de iudiciis et cautelis *cyroycorum* (cyrurgicorum), quod in certis casibus et maxime in fractura cranei *necesse* prodest, *uti* et sunt decem notabilia sive indicia. (Capitulum VI)

Nam (Iam) ad hoc quod de fractura cranei verum vel falsum cognoscatur, et ut ostendat cyrurgicus quod sit ingeniosus artifex *cyrurgicus*, et plusquam perfectus, et integer[e] inter ceteros magis

of the stomach, the humors course to the stomach from sympathy and impedes the rising of fumes to the head. Should the patient insist on drinking wine, let him drink weak, dilute ordinary valley wine to which is added hot water and a little sugar. This is known as "sour wine"[85] and contains twice as much water as wine.

The diet for those who do not have fractured skulls but merely wounds of the skin and galea[86] is restricted to the above until the eighth day, at which time the patient is secure from the danger of hot pus. Thereafter, return to the necessary and usual principles contained in a previous section. Note that in cases of fractured skulls or lacerated heads all practicing physicians use rose oil and rose honey and do good therewith.

Chapter VI

Section concerning advice and cautions for surgeons in certain situations, especially for skull fractures, presented in the form of ten hints or notations.

---

[85]vinum ponticum
[86]almocanti

appereat, atque de sua operatione ea quae sunt archana (humane) nature *et sibi ventuta circum circa aspicientibus clare notescat* (cognoscat, ea que sequuntur optime memorie mandet). Sed per hoc ea quae sunt infra, nota sunt inventa ut pauper cyrurgicus citius extirpet pecuniam iam diu acquisitam sine postulatione ex suo labore cum benivolentia captanda, et maxime de manibus ingratorum qui non *cupiunt eritare servitium a medico illatum* (volunt satisfacere servitio a medico accepto) nisi postquam medicus *contrariaverit ad ea quae fecit vel* (opposuerit eis de eo quod) facere potest mala fortuna. Nam cum *tibi primo* (primum) occurrit *aliquam lesionem* alique lesio) a causa primitiva in capite factam, aut a casu *aut ab* (et) offensione de qua forte ignorabis cranei fracturam, (hoc tibi inferius) ex decem modis apparebit per signa *empirica* (specifica) facta ad *exteriora* (extra), et aliquando erronea in *aliquibus* (certis) casibus, et longa a via veritatis, sed cum (his) iudiciis et cautelis inferius tangendis satis veritas *bene intelligendo* (intelligendo) cum effectu *et non cum defectu* experiri potest. Et ista maxime fiant *a* cyrurgico cum in loco *et ordine* et in vulnere convenienti sufficiens apparebit tempus et maxime quando aliquis amicus vel attinens infirmus *super hoc* fuerit, et *ygnorams et ygnoraverit* (ignorabis seu dubitabis de cranei fractura), quoniam vivere cautelose (et) cautela saepe prodest (Galienus).

Sequitur de primo iudicio et de prima cautela cyroycorum.

Primum ergo iudicium in iudicando de fractura cranei sit *tibi notum* (hoc). Sunt (nota) aliqui qui *bipedalem* (longam duorum pedum) c[h]ordam *heream* (eream) vel *calibicis* (calibis) accipiunt *monacord* (monocordi seu salterii), et unam extremitatem *accipiunt* (capiunt) cum duobus dentibus taliter, ne c[h]orda contangatur a labiis infirmi. Alter *a vero* (autem) extremitas c[h]ordae circumvoluatur [76r] *in police* (polici) et foriter extendatur, sicut fit in *monacordo* (monocordo) *simphonie* (sinfoniae). Sed cum altera *vero* manu (vel) infirmi, et hoc *maxime* (modo) *cum uno digito* fiat tintinatio. Nam si[c] vox melodiae rauc[h]a *est* ad craneum fractum ascendat, tunc af[f]irmant ubi dicit eger sensisse talem sonitum obtusum in capite ibidem esse fracturam.

Secundum iudicium ad iudicandum *adhuc* de fractura cranei est tale. Nam adhuc sunt aliqui *fialam* (tubam) habentes et *egrum* facientes o[b]tuse in ipsam suf[f]lare ut tubator in tuba tubante taliter ut (spiritus seu) flatus sursum ad craneum ascendat. Si autem *aer* (eger) ad extra craneum per vulnus ex tali suf[f]latione respiret hec est talis sufflatio, est signum fracture cranei manifestum.

Since the diagnosis of skull fractures is uncertain, the following is presented, so that the surgeon may show his skill and superiority, when compared to other physicians, and that he may know the operations of those things secret to human nature. Let him commit the following to memory. From what is given below, remarks are devised to enable the poor surgeon quickly to obtain his fees for his labor with grateful payment, as in former times, without haggling, especially from the hands of ingrates who do not want to settle up unless the physician administer something which does them harm. In the beginning of an illness, when a lesion occurs in the head from a primary cause either from misfortune or accident, and if you are uncertain whether a skull fracture is present, this will become apparent to you in the following ten ways, through specific external signs. Although you may err in certain respects and be a long way from the truth, with the signs and cautions given below, the truth can be intelligently and effectively arrived at. These diagnostic tests the surgeon performs when the time appears right in the site and in the wound and especialy when either friend or family be sick and you are uncertain about the presence of a skull fracture. For, "To live by caution is often profitable". Galen.

The first sign, therefore, in advising concerning fractured skulls is this: Some take a 2 foot music string from a monochord or a saltery and bind one end to two teeth, insuring that the string does not touch the patient's lips. Tie [76^{r}] the other end to the tip of the patient's thumb and pluck the string vigorously, as one does to produce a resonant note.[87] If, however, a discord ensues in the patient, the raucous melody has risen to a fractured skull. Determine where in his head the patient feels such dull sounds, and at that point is the fracture.

The second sign. There are some who have horns and they bid the patient blow, as a trumpeter blows his horn, so that the spirit or wind rises up to the patient's head. If the air from this blowing respires to the exterior of the wound, this is a manifest sign of a fractured skull.

The third sign. There are some who bid the patient chew hard beans, hazel nuts or other nuts. If pain is felt or the sound of cracked nuts resound throughout the patient's head, this indicates a cranial fracture.

The fourth valuable sign in occult skull fractures. There are those who place the handle of a knife or hard wood, etc., between

[87]monochordo singonio

Tertium iudicium *adhuc* ad iudicandum de fractura cranei *est tale*. Nam *adhuc* sunt aliqui qui fabam duram masticare *faciunt* vel avellanas *sive* (vel) nuces *vel consimiles egrotanti* (egro) frangere iubent, et si dolor sive sonitus fracturae talium nucum fractarum *si sit aliquid quod tristem rei sensationem in loco offenso fecerit dicunt fractura ibidem fractura cranei esse signum manifestum* (pervenerit ipsi craneo tunc iudicant de fractura cranei.)

Quartum iudicium *adhuc* estimativum de fractura cranei occulta *sit tale*. *Nam adhuc* sunt (nota) aliqui qui manubrium cultelli, sive lignum durum vel consimile ponendo inter dentes infirmi, et constringendo hoc tale seriatim, et procedendo ab uno capite (duorum) dentium usque ad aliud caput mandibule. Si vero os cranei fuerit fractum erit dolor in loco offenso quod est rationabile et consonum, et hoc est propter colligantiam sive communitatem panniculorum sub craneo positorum ad ipsum dentem actu facientem dolorem in tali constrictione mediante suo nervo *et illo* denti *descendente* (descendenti), quod manifestum esse potest in anothomia cuiuslibet dentis, et hoc est, quia omnis dens habet foramen in radice in quo dente *pertransit* nervus sensitivus ad ipsum dentem. Sed hec est causa, *quia dens multum dolet. Rerum non propter ipsum dentem. Ratio quia ossa non dolent* (quia dentes multum colent non per se ipsos et cetera, quia ossa non dolent). Sed (dicuntur) dolere propter nervum ad ipsum venientem, et dentem cum gingiva ligantem.

Quintum iudicium *adhuc* de fractura cranei occulat, et non *bene* nota *est tale*. Nam sunt aliqui volentes scire de fractura cranei manifesta, et tamen *superficialis* (superficialiter) *apparens* (apparente) utrum penetret ad utrumque latus vel non transeat meditullium, id est medietatem inclusive *vel exclusive* ipsius ossis cranei. Et isti tales super orificio ossis fracti ponunt *cotum* (bombicem) carminatum modicum, et iubent *quod infirmus* (infirmum) cum sua manu recta, (ut) o[b]turet suum os cum naribus suf[f]lando tamdiu donec flatus sursum ascendat, et si *bonbax* (bombix) aliqualiter) moveatur *a fractura*, tunc est signum manifeste penetrationis. Et aliquando si penetrat talis fractura sic suf[f]lando dura mater elevatur, et humiditatem intrinsecam ad extra expellendo, (ita quod) omnibus aspicientibus manifeste patet.

Sextum iudicium in iudicando de fractura *cranei sit tale*. Nam multotiens accidit *ut* concava pars cranei (ut) versus cerebrum frangatur absque *convessa* (convexa), quae est pars versus al-

the teeth of the patient and bind up the teeth in series from the crown of one on the maxillary side to the crown of the opposite on the mandible. If the skull is fractured, pain will appear at the site of injury. This is understandable and consistent, since the ligaments or the companions of the periosteum placed under the skull transmit sharp pain to the occluded tooth through the mediation of the descending nerve to the tooth. This can be verified from the dental anatomy, for all teeth have foramina in their roots through which a sensory nerve enters. This is why teeth ache; it is not [from the teeth] themselves, for bone is insensitive. They are said to hurt because of nerves coursing to the bone and the teeth, which are connected to the gums.

The fifth sign hitherto unrecognized concerning occult skull fracture. In desiring to learn whether a seemingly superficial skull fracture penetrates the diploë enclosed in the interior of the skull bone, there are some who place over the hole of the fractured skull a small piece of carmine [stained] cotton. They then have the patient squeeze his nostrils with his right hand, bidding him blow through his nose until the breath rises to the surface. If the cotton moves in any way from the fracture, this is a manifest sign of penetration. Sometimes when the fracture penetrates, this blowing elevates the dura mater and the intrinsic humors are expelled to the outside. This is obvious from all appearances.

The sixth sign. It often happens that the concave part of the bone facing the brain is fractured, but not the convexity which faces the galea.[86] This can occur when missiles are fired or stones thrown. These pierce the tables, resulting in the fracture of the inner table without involvement of the outer part. But the astute physician will well identify this, inspecting carefully the region above to determine if it be denuded or uncovered. In the middle, visible superficially, dark or dusky blood will often appear, which nature transports to this place in order to reach the affected part. This is the putrid blood discharge[88] or the pus of putrefication. Unless it is quickly removed with the expirator, it has a bad import. [76v]

Seventh sign. Often the fracture extends just to the middle table of the skull, removing some superficial bone. In the skull defect great pulsations appear, and you may not appreciate the

---

[88]humiditas sanguinea putrida

mocatim, sicut patere potest de *lapide falare sive* (de falaria, sive de lapide) *bonbarde* (bombarde) in muro *poriecto* (proiecta). Nam pars intrinseca muri rimulatur *fortiter* (maxime) absque parte extrinseca, sed ad hoc *ut* medicus *astutus* (bene acutus) istud bene *cognoscat* (cognoscet) aspirciat super os si erit denudatum, sive discoopertum (et) acute (prospiciat), quia in *meditulio* (meditulo) ap[p]arebit per transparentiam partis *superficialis* (superficialiter) *quendam oppacum* (quidam opacus) sive *fuscum* (fuscus) *sanguinem* (sanguis) quem natura ibidem transmisit propter *partem offensam subvenire* (ut parti offense subveniat), et hic est humiditas sanguinea putrida, sive apta putrefieri cum malis accidentibus, nisi cito subveniat(ur) cum *expiraculo* (expiraclatio). [76v]

Septium (Aliud) iudicium *adhuc* de fractura cranei *sit tale*. Nam saepe contingit craneum frangi usque ad meditullium, et non ultra, et aliqua pars *superficialis* (superficialiter) ossis fuerit remota, et in foramine ossis fracti contingit fieri maxima pulsatio, et *per* (super) hoc non iudices talem motum esse cerebri si anothomiam illius membri ignorabis. Nam per *medirallium* (meditulium) intelligere debemus porositates existentes in medio sive in superficiebus concavi et *convessi* (conveni) ipsius ossis cranei, ad quas porositates sive duas inter tabulas *secundam aliquos* seminate sunt venae pulsatiles, et ipsum os nutrientes atque motum, sicut cerebrum habentes propter arteriarum desiderium eventationis.

Octavum (Aliud) iudicium ad iudicandum de s[c]issura rimulari in craneo. *Nam* quia saepe contingit s[c]isura[m] rimularem fieri in craneo, et ad oculum manifeste non apparere, quia per unum certum iudicium a cyrurgico extimativum *apprehendi* (comprehendi) potest. Iudicium autem est tale. Nam sunt aliqui qui *capiunt* (accipiunt) *enclaustrum* (incaustrum) scriptorum ad ignem calefactum, et inhibunt stuelos in ipso *enclaustro* (incaustro) qui debent poni super partem discoopertam cranei de qua parte cranei lesa cum s[c]issura[m] dubitas esse *superficialis* (superficialem) vel profunda[m], et sic *dimictis* (dimittis) stuel*l*os *inhibitas* per spatium (spacium) unius mutationis vel donec *enclaustrum* (inclaustrum) in s[c]issura *exsiccatum* (exiccatum) fuerit quod *enclaustrum* (incaustrum) si in s[c]issura fuerit tergi non poterit donec (usque) ad finem *raspando cum raspatorio* (veniens) amplius nigredo sequens s[c]issuram videri non poterit et sic in *secunda* (cum alia) mutatione *iterum reitera* (reiteret) cum *inpositione* (inponitione) *enclaustrum* (incaustri) vel alterius liquoris donec de fine s[c]issure *eris* (fueris) bene certificatus.

brain movement unless you understand the anatomy of that structure. For around the middle table one should know that holes exist in the middle between concavity and convexity of the skull. Between these two tables run pulsating veins nourishing the bone. The cerebrum has motion because of these arteries, in consideration of its need for ventilation.[89]

Eighth sign concerning linear skull fracture.[90] It often happens that a linear skull fracture, invisible to the eye, can be established by the examining surgeon through one certain sign. This is the sign: there are those who soak wicks in hot caustics, mentioned in the literature, and place them above the injured part of the head when they are uncertain whether the lesion is superficial or deep. The wicks are changed one or more times, until the caustic is removed in the linear fracture, for if the caustic is beneath the fracture site it will not be cleansed away until discharge no longer comes up through the fissure. The wicks are soaked with caustic or other liquors several times until the extent of the fissure is ascertained.

Ninth obvious, defensible and prudent counsel. When a large part of the skull is removed, take care lest air enter the brain. There are, for example, some physicians, who, when confronted with a situation where a large skull fracture exists and where great portions of the bone have been removed or will be removed in stages because of the comminution, fear that the wick or plaster may compress the dura mater, causing harm to the brain from pressure or extrinsic air. In these instances they take part of a gourd, shape it to the form of the rent and cover the skull defect. This is done for four reasons: First, that the laymen marvel at such a solid covering, for they take the part of the cup in the head of others to be a solid covering; this is erroneous and impossible. Second, lest vapor enter a skull defect without a head plaster. Third, lest compression be caused by the ligatures; and last, that the discharge under the bone more easily escape without the compression of heavy objects. Insure that the cup has many holes.

Tenth sign concerns the approach of certain death. Note that when misfortune occurs and a head lesion ensues, whatever kind it be, whether with a wound or visible fracture, the following signs

[89]eventatio
[90]scissure rimulare

Nonum (Aliud) iudicium visibile defensorium et cautelosum ad evitandum, ne aer ingrediatur in cerebro ubi fuerit magna remotio partis ossis. Sunt aliqui pra[c]ticantes per hunc modum exempli gratia, (ponatur) quod sit magna ossis fractura in capite, et maxima pars ossis remota vel removibilis propter multa paulatine *frustra* (frusta) sed timendo ne stuelli cum explastro conprimant duram matrem et cerebrum (conturbet) in suis oppositionibus, et ipsum (cerebrum) cum aere extrinseco inpediatur. *Nam* in hoc *communi* casu *asignato* accipiunt, et *bene* (optime) faciunt, unam partem cucurbitae ad formam coopertorii, et foramen cranei cooperiunt, et hoc fieri potest propter quatuor causas. Prima causa ut *stoycus* (stolidum) vulgus admiretur de tali consolidatione, qui dicunt *se vidisse* partem cucurbitae in cap*i*tibus aliquorum esse consolidatam, quod est falsum, et impossibile. *Secunda causa* (Secundo modi) fieri potest ne aer in foramine cranei absque emplastro capitali ingrediatur. Tertia causa fieri potest ne compressio fiat per ligaturas et revolutiones multas ligaturae quae fiunt in capite ips*am* cucurbit*am* *sublevando* (sublevante) ligaturam. *Quatua* (Alia) causa *fieri potest* est ut sanies de sub osse melius expurgari possit, sine compressione rerum gravantium, *at* (sed) tamen debent esse multa foramina existentia in ipsa cucurbita.

Decimum iudicium et sententia mortalis de proximo et absque dubio sit tale (Aliud iudicium de propinquo adventu mortis absque dubio). Nota quod quando adfuerit casus et offensio superveniens in capite et quomodocumque fiat *sive* (sine) fuerit cum vulnere, sive cum fractura, (sive) apparens, sive non, et pulsus fuerit inequalis sive inordinatus, et forte fuerit febris lenta vel magna, aut vigiliae et inquietudines, et vomitus sive [77^{r}] subversio, *aut* (et) alienatio mentis sive permixtio rationis et appetitus fuerit prostratus ad sumendum cibum et potum, vel fuerit *aliquod signum* (aliquid signorum) saltem istorum usque ad septimum diem, et si ultra haec (signa) *supra assignata persevereaverint: iudica craneum esse fractum*, etiam apostema in panniculis esse factum, quod est signum mortis in brevi, nisi cito *subcurratur* (succurratur) cum modis *et temporibus.*

may appear up to the seventh day: unequal or irregular[91] pulse, elevated or persistent fever, wakefulness and restlessness, vomiting [77r] or retching, delirium,[92] confusion, and loss of appetite. If any of these foregoing signs persist beyond this day, the diagnosis is that of a skull fracture accompanied by pus of the membranes. This is a herald of death unless the condition be cured quickly by the methods touched upon.

---

[91]inordinatus
[92]alienato mentis

IV

Commentary on Leonard of Bertapaglia's *On Skull Fractures*

Chapter I of the *De Fractura Cranei* [68^v] begins with a preface. Leonard chose to insert it in the section on skull fractures rather than at the beginning of the *Cyrurgia*, as with Theodoric,[1] for example, and we are justified in regarding this as attestation to Leonard's stress on the nervous system. The work is addressed to his son, Fabricius, "a lad of eleven years," a form of dedication used by Chaucer and others.[2]

In his preface, Leonard promises to "follow another method not adopted from my predecessor, citing diverse sources. . ." This may refer either to the list of authorities paraded in Chapter IV or, more probably, to the case report given in Chapter III. In fact, the special case report was not unknown to Leonard's predecessors. The Hippocratic physicians in the *Epidemics*[3] present case studies, as does Rhazes.[4,5] Other medieval authors, such as Lisfranc,[6] also describe patients observed or treated, but Leonard's special chapter is unique.

Before proceeding with the examination of the text, we should delineate the neurosurgical domain as it existed in the fifteenth century. With regard to epilepsy, Hippocratic physicians[7] had rec-

[1] *The Surgery of Theodoric*, Trans. Eldridge Campbell and James Colton. (New York, 1955–1960), vol. 1, pp. 3–7.

[2] William of Saliceto dedicated his work to his son, Bernardinus; see Benedict, *Handbuch der Algemeinen Chirurgie*. (Breslau, 1842), p. 5.

[3] Hippocrates, *Epidemics* III.13.

[4] Owsei Temkin, "A Medieval Translation of Rhazes' Clinical Observations." *Bull. Hist. Med. 12:*102, 1942.

[5] L. M. Sadi, "The Millenium of Ar-Razi (Rhazes)." *Ann. Med. Hist. 7:*63, 1935.

[6] Lisfranc, Tract. 1, Cap. 2. *Cyrurgia Parva Lanfranci*, in *Cyrurgia Guidonis de Cauliaco*. (Venice, 1498, *Collectio Cyrurgia Veneta*)

[7] Hippocrates, *On the Sacred Disease* 2.11.

ommended medical treatment but surgical inroads had been made early in the Middle Ages, as the Bamberg Surgery fragments attest.[8] By the fifteenth century, however, the practice of trepanation for epilepsy had waned.[9] Surgery for hydrocephalus[10,11] likewise had been all but abandoned by the fifteenth century, although ventricular tap had been used as late as the time of Guy de Chauliac. With regard to psychosurgery, Theodoric[12] performed surgery in an effort to restore memory while Roger is said to have recommended trepanation for insanity.[13] Notwithstanding, neither indication was generally accepted in Leonard's time so that head trauma remained the chief indication for surgical intervention.

The author begins his text on skull fractures [68ᵛ] by offering eight requirements for becoming a good surgeon. Once again, Leonard assigned this subject to the nervous system, rather than as in the *Chyrurgia* of Guy de Chauliac to the beginning of the text. The "condition," or requirements were a popular subject throughout the Middle Ages. Leonard's prerequisites differ little from those of Guy de Chauliac,[14] who had enjoyed greater popularity. But other variations are known, contained in the works of Isaac Judaeus,[15] St. Jerome, and others. MacKinney[16] has shown in his excellent study that the format of the prerequisites derives from an amalgam of the Hippocratic *Art* and the *Oath*, gradually evolving into what later came to be known as the prerequisites for the good surgeon.

Compared with the clarity and simplicity of Guy de Chauliac, Leonard's advice seems inelegant but, notwithstanding, has certain compelling qualities. Leonard cautions the student not to refuse a fee, not to haggle over payment, and encourages frank discussion between patient and physician. This advice from an academician

---

[8]George W. Corner, "Bamberg Surgery." *Bull. Inst. Hist. Med. 5:*1–32, 1937.

[9]See Theodoric, Book IV.9.

[10]Guy de Chauliac, . . . Tract. 2, Doc. 2, Cap. 1.

[11]Antoine Portal, *Histoire de l'Anatomie et de la Chirurgie.* (Paris, 1770), vol. 1, p. 185.

[12]Theodoric, Book 2, chapter 2; Cecilia C. Mettler, *History of Medicine* (Philadelphia, 1947), p. 833, is in error.

[13]Roger, I.26.

[14]Guy de Chauliac, *Capitulum Universale*, or Tract. 1, Doc. 1, Cap. 1.

[15]Saul Jarcho, "Guide for Physicians (Musar Harofim) by Isaac Judaeus (880–932)." *Bull. Hist. Med. 15:*180, 1944.

[16]Loren C. MacKinney, "Medical Ethics and Etiquette in the Early Middle Ages: The Persistence of Hippocratic Ideals." *Bull. Hist. Med. 26:*1, 1952.

and a highly successful practitioner affords us insight into his contemporary fame and public esteem. Other physicians had a more aggressive posture: "The more you demand for your services and the higher you set your fee, the more your work will be respected by the public."[17] But Leonard is no milksop about the matter of remuneration and elsewhere we see that he does not dismiss the practice of giving the intransigent patient a dose of salts if he does not pay up. The approximate fee for a visit was about 10 solida,[18] subject to the usual adjustment to the patient's financial means. One physician refused to attend the Pope unless his fee was assured in advance![19] The annual fee for a lecturer in surgery was about 100 lire,[20] but it is not likely that Leonard depended too heavily on this for income.

In characteristic fashion, Leonard interrupts his discussion of the requirements for a good surgeon to describe a case he treated [68^v]. A patient had sustained a comminuted skull fracture and Leonard succeeded in painlessly removing a piece of bone with a secret instrument made of parchment. The nature of his instrument cannot be easily determined; perhaps it was a kind of lenticular. If so, the fragment must have been loose. Leonard is not lavish with his descriptions of technique, for this was a matter to be taught the student by his master during the preceptorship, that is to say, between the bachelor's degree and licentiate. Furthermore, defending charges of braggadocio, Leonard cites three witnesses to this surgery: two famous medical colleagues[21] and one barber surgeon. Much has been prated of the implacable hatred between the short and long gowns—barbers and surgeons—but here we have evidence of easy communication between the two schools.

Chapter II [69^r] begins by recounting eleven items of importance in the treatment of skull fracture. Medieval surgeons identified seven skull bones: two parietal, two temporal, one frontal

---

[17]Jarcho, ref. 15.

[18]Theodor Puschmann, *A History of Medical Education*, Trans E. H. Hare. (London, 1891), p. 277. The tuition fee for a medical student was 20 solidi; Lynn Thorndike, *University Records and Life in the Middle Ages*. (New York, 1944), p. 384.

[19]David Riesman, *The Story of Medicine in the Middle Ages*. (New York, 1935), p. 94.

[20]Thorndike, ref. 18, p. 368.

[21]One of the witnesses was Marsilius de Santa Sophia, who also had composed a commentary on the Fourth Canon. In other words, he gave the same course. Lynn Thorndike, "Some later Medieval Latin Medical Manuscripts at Berne and Prague." *Ann. Med. Hist. N.S. 8:*427, 1936.

(called coronal, including the nasal and orbital bones), one occipital and the sphenoid "basilar bones."[22,23] Guy de Chauliac[24] criticized William of Salicet and Lisfranc for faulty notions about the basilar skull. The basilar bones also included the crista galli, but this structure was considered unimportant.[25]

The eleven notations begin with a caution to prevent pus formation. Leonard lists cold as the primary cause of pus, resting on an unbroken chain of tradition from the time of the Greco-Roman school to Avicenna.[26]

The second cause is a depressed skull fracture. Leonard cites the authority of Avicenna[27] in recommending that depressed bone fragments be removed. Actually, two schools had evolved. Theodoric and Hugo[28] were conservative; they did not enlarge the wound or remove a fragment "with force," i.e., they removed only loose fragments. Earlier, nonintervention also had been the practice in Padua, as Guy de Chauliac reported.[29] Opposed to this was the aggressive school,[30] Guy de Chauliac concurring, which recommended "dilating" (enlarging) the wound and removing the depressed fragment. The surgeon accomplished this by boring a series of holes around the depressed fragment. He then lifted it up with an elevator.[31] (Leonard, moreover, had a unique instrument called the *moicula*, to be discussed below.) Leonard wisely cautions against permitting the tent or drain to cause pressure over the skull defect, lest the brain be injured.

Another cause of pus [69^{v}] is an improper regimen and a plethora of humors. Again, the author cites the merits of phlebotomy, a method of general evacuation whereby redundant humors widely distributed throughout the body are eliminated.

The third remark warns the physician about concerning him-

---

[22]Thomas Louth, *Histoire de l'Anatomie.* (Strasburg, 1815), vol. 1, p. 205.

[23]Karl Sudhoff, *Studien zur Geschichte der Medizin 4:*34, 1908, who prints a Dresden MS. of 1323.

[24]Guy de Chauliac, Tract. 1, Doc. 2, Cap. 1.

[25]Celsus, *De Medicina* II.8.40.

[26]Avicenna, Canon 4, Fen 5, Tract. 3, Cap. 1; Canon 1.

[27]Avicenna, Canon 4, Fen 5, Tract. 3, Cap. 1.

[28]N. Kjaergaard, *Om Drainagen in den aeldre chirurgi.* (Copenhagen, 1892), p. 96.

[29]Guy de Chauliac, Tract. 3, Doc. 2, Cap. 1.

[30]The Four Masters give the indications for surgery of depressed skull fractures: if a fragment lodges under healthy bone; if a fragment pierces the dura mater; and if a "tumor" appears in the wound. (I.3).

[31]Lisfranc, II.1, *op.cit.,* ref. 6.

self solely with the skull fracture, ignoring the general complexity of the problem. He lists the untoward symptoms that might result. The fourth remark recommends that the physician ought not remove all the fragments, but only those that are depressed and detached, since they will not heal. This is still regarded as sound surgical advice.

Leonard alludes to the membranes of the brain [69ᵛ]. In the early treatises, the word *siphac* was used for both meninges and peritoneum, but later authors substituted *mirac* for peritoneum, reserving the term *siphac* for meninges.[32,33] Two of the coverings, the *dura mater* and the *pia mater*, were identified and named after their gross characteristics. The pia embraces the soft brain and, therefore, was teleologically soft. Its function is to protect the brain against shock waves.[34] The dura is coarse because it is adjacent to bone. The ancients recognized that the dura mater adhered to the sutures of the skull and was continuous with the pericranium,[35] and that the pia mater provided vascular nourishment for the brain.

In the fifth remark [69ᵛ], Leonard discusses prognostication. The substance of his remarks is only a fragment of what was then taught about the subject. Reference might be made to Guy de Chauliac's analysis,[36] for example, which was considerably more sophisticated. Leonard states that if the membranes are lacerated, then orbital erythema, pain, orificial discharge, obtundation, and vomiting ensue. If reason is lost, the lesion is anterior; with impaired memory, the lesion is posterior. Contralaterality of the lesion to motor-sensory symptoms was, of course, well established[37] in his day.

Leonard notes in his sixth remark that skull fractures differ from other fractures. That they were more dangerous had universal agreement: *Judicia fractura cranei est periculose apud omnes*.[38]

---

[32]Avicenna, Canon 3, Fen 1, Tract. 1, Cap. 1.

[33]Guy de Chauliac, Tract. 1, Doc. 2, Cap. 1.

[34]Galen, *De Usu Partium* VIII.9: Et porro ipsius tegmentum et crassa meninx aut potius non simpliciter ipsam tegumentum nominare oportet, sed magis velut perpugnaculum quodam propulsandis cranii impressionibus oppositum.

[35]Guy de Chauliac, Tract. 1, Doc. 2, Cap. 1: dura matre origitur per commissura pericranium a pia matre infunditur cerebro nutrementum.

[36]Guy de Chauliac, Tract. 3, Doc. 2, Cap. 1.

[37]*Ibid.*: Et in vulneribus perveniectibus ad panniculum cerebri accidit lixatas in latere volneris et spasmus in opposito.

[38]Guy de Chauliac, Tract. 3, Doc. 2, Cap. 1: "Judgment about skull fractures is hazardous for everybody."

Moreover, the mechanisms of fracture[39] and the distinctive qualities of the skull were important factors to be considered. Medieval surgeons attributed the porosity of the cranium to the teleologic necessity for lightness (Galen).[40] The roundness which Leonard mentions has two purposes: to increase skull capacity and to decrease vulnerability to trauma (Avicenna[41] and Mondinus[42]). Avicenna further observed that callus (*arosboth*) does not form in a skull fracture,[43] because the skull is membranous bone.

The seventh remark relates to surgical technique. Where should the incision be placed? Leonard offers competent and unmistakably practical advice. Be direct, place your incision over the depressed bone and avoid nerves, he counsels the student. Guy de Chauliac[44] also adds: work quickly, avoid surgery on debilitated patients. Other surgeons recommend stuffing cotton into the patient's ear so that he would not hear the noise,[45] bone conduction notwithstanding. The practice persists down to the present day. The Four Masters[46] also caution about cutting the superficial temporal artery, a most troublesome vessel.

In the eighth notation, Leonard repeats Avicenna's caution against procrastinating too long before surgery. Attention is invited to Leonard's use of the word *sanies* [70^r], which I have variously translated as "discharge" or retained the original *sanies*. Others might have preferred *superflues*, used in early English medical texts. *Sanies* has been defined by Avicenna[47] as a body fluid that cannot be converted to the four primary humors and, hence, cannot be transformed into actual body substances. It must, therefore, be expelled.

Ninth, the author describes the appropriate treatment for a gangrenous discharge (*nigredo*). He affirms the appearance of nigredo to be a bad prognostic sign. The tenth remark [70^v] concerns

---

[39]Charles Daremberg, *Glossulae Quatuor Magistrorum super Chirurgiam Rogerii et Rolandi*. (Paris, 1854), Book 1, Cap. 7.

[40]Galen, *De Usu Partium* IX.2.

[41]Avicenna, Canon 1, Fen 1, Doc. 5, Summa 1, Cap. 2.

[42]C. A. E. Wickersheimer, *Anatomies de Mondino dei Luzzi*. (Paris, 1926), pp. 40–41.

[43]Avicenna, Canon 4, Fen 5, Tract. 3, Cap. 1.

[44]Guy de Chauliac, Tract. 3, Doc. 2, Cap. 1.

[45]Theodoric II.6; Avicenna, Canon 4, Fen 5, Tract. 3, Cap. 1.

[46]Daremberg, ref. 39, Book 1, Cap. 1: Quando sit vulnus in anterioribus partibus cranei versus tempora, difficilis est curationis propter abscicionem arterie.

[47]Avicenna, Canon 1, Fen 1, Tract. 4.

the use of the cautery in head wounds. Leonard alludes to the iron cautery. Metal was used,[48] of course, so that the instrument when heated would occlude the blood vessels, much the same as the modern electric cautery seals off bleeding vessels. Boiling oil, however, was preferred by Leonard and later medieval surgeons for hemostasis. Either way, the purpose was, according to Guy de Chauliac,[49] to comfort the membrane, protect from corruption, stop blood flow, and purge and attract the discharges. In the eleventh notation, Leonard discusses the use of topical medications.

Chapter III [70^{v}] begins with the recounting of a story within a story. A peasant, whose nephew had previously been treated for knife wounds, was brought to Leonard. Characteristically, Leonard first tells us about the nephew, who had had multiple lacerations: one in the hepatic flexure with resultant fistula, the second in the chest cavity, and the third in the subcostal area. More to the point, the uncle had a spear wound which penetrated the brain substance of the frontal region, involving the lateral ventricle. In this connection Leonard quotes Galen, who had described at least two cases of brain injury often cited by medieval physicians. Although Leonard alludes to the illustration in the *Aphorisms*, he might have more appropriately used the case mentioned in the *De Usu Partium*,[50] since the former describes a wound of the grey matter, whereas in the latter the ventricle was involved. Galen's description in the *De Usu Partium* reads: "We have seen in Smyrnia in Ionia a marvelous thing. We have seen a young man, injured in one of the ventricles, survive the accident because of, as it seemed, the grace of God." The Four Masters[51] had no such experience. Arnold of Villanova[52] treated a brain injury and Guy de Chauliac[53] reported a wound of the posterior brain with recovery. Moreover, Guy de Chauliac distinguishes between a simple wound of the grey matter and a wound with brain swelling and consequent *fungus cerebri*, i.e., herniation

---

[48]See discussion in Guy de Chauliac, Tract. 4, Doc. 4.

[49]Guy de Chauliac, Tract. 3, Doc. 2, Cap. 1.

[50]Galen, *De Usu Partium* VIII.10: Nam admirabile illud spectaculum aliquam incredibile quod Smyrnem in Ionia accidit; aliquando sumus conspicate adolescentum vulnere in alterum anteriorum ventriculorum accepto, superstitem fuisse dei voluntate.

[51]Daremberg, ref. 39, Book 1, Ch. 1: Si autem fiat vulnus in contumatia capitis: ad substantiam cerebri transent vel procedat mortal est.

[52]Cited by Leonard in chapter 3 of the *De Fractura Cranei*.

[53]Guy de Chauliac, Tract. 3, Doc. 1, Cap. 1 quotes two cases of Galen.

through the skull opening. This distinction Leonard also makes. Leonard undertook treatment of the uncle and demonstrated his patient to "many doctors and scholars of Padua whom I enticed there with prayers and entreaties." Apparently Leonard was too much of a pedagogue to miss an opportunity to demonstrate a patient with cerebrospinal fistula and *fungus cerebri*. Clinical demonstrations were not unusual in Padua, for Tassignano also exhibited interesting cases.[54]

Apparently Leonard's patients did well for a month, whereupon posttraumatic seizures supervened, followed by contralateral paralysis (abscess?). The outcome, although not stated, may be presumed attributed entirely, of course, to the patient's failure to heed his surgeon's advice.

The medieval physician divided the ventricles into three compartments. The two anterior ventricles [70ᵛ], or lateral ventricles as they are known today, were regarded as the seat of imagination and each was called the *cellula phantasica*; the third ventricle, where reason resided, was termed the *cellula logistica*; while the fourth ventricle, the *cellula memorialis*, was the repository of memory. Guy de Chauliac explained that the ancients compared the ventricles to the three chambers of the temple. In the first, declarations were made; in the second, statements shifted; and in the third, final sentence pronounced. Accordingly, we gather information in the first, reflect in the second, and formulate in the third. This concept finds almost universal support in the medieval literature (Galen,[55] Avicenna,[56] Lisfranc,[57] and Niccolus Physicus[58]).

The ventricles had added importance according to the school of Erasistratus. Air absorbed by the lungs is transformed by the heart into the vital spirit and dispatched to the body and brain. Once in the brain, it is carried to the ventricle where it is converted into the animal spirit and then conveyed throughout the body by the hollow nerves. The Galenic system differed in several respects. The *rete mirabilis* (Circle of Willis) usurped the function of the ventricular system as the location of the animal spirit. In the Galenic

[54]Lynn Thorndike, *Science and Thought in the Fifteenth Century*. (New York and London, 1963), p. 104.

[55]Galen, *De Usu Partium* VIII.9.

[56]Avicenna, Canon 3, Fen 1, Tract. 1, Cap. 2.

[57]Lisfranc II.2.

[58]George Washington Corner, *Anatomical Texts of the Earlier Middle Ages*. (Washington, 1927), p. 71.

system, chyle from the intestines is sent by way of the portal vein to the liver. There it is transformed into the natural (or nutritive) spirit. Thence it is dispatched to the heart, where it enters from the right chamber through a small interventricular septum into the left side. Here it mixes with the pneuma from the lungs brought to the heart by the pulmonary vein to form the vital spirit. This is sent to the brain by way of the *rete mirabili* to form the animal spirit. Thus, Erasistratus identifies two spirits to Galen's three.[59] Leonard accepts three spirits, of course, to accord with Galenic tradition.

In the closing paragraph of Chapter III, reference is made to the critical days. If the patient with a brain injury survived seven days, it was believed that the chances for recovery were good.[60] How bitter Leonard's disappointment, in the case of the uncle cited in the third chapter, to encounter posttraumatic complications one month following injury. And this in a case exhibited to his medical colleagues, presumably when the patient had been doing well.

Leonard calls the fourth chapter [71^{v}] the "theoretical chapter." Avicenna defines the theoretical consideration as "that which, when mastered, gives us a certain kind of knowledge apart from any question of treatment."[61] Leonard begins by citing authority. His range is impressive. It includes Aesculapius, Anaxogaras, Constantinius Viaticus, the sect of Thessaly,[62] Hippocrates, Galen, Avicenna, Peter Abano (Conciliator), William of Verignana (Gulielmus de Vergnoza, Bolognese physician, *c.* 1333), Gerard of Gordon (Lilius Gordonsis de Pedmont),[63] Bruno Longoburgo of Padua, Theodoric of Cervia, Erasistratus (Epistropes), Arnold of Villanova, Philagrius[64] (Plorigerus), Roger of Parma (Ruggiero), Lanfrachi (Alafrancus), Albertus Magnus, Peter Argelata (Anagellatus), Peter of Ussignana (Trusiano), Francis of Pedemont (14th

[59]Charles Joseph Singer, *The Evolution of Anatomy*. (London, 1925), pp. 31–82.

[60]Galen defends the critical days in his *On the Natural Faculties* I.14. In general, the 7th, 19th, 21st, and 28th days of the moon are favorable. See Reisman, ref. 19, p. 98.

[61]Avicenna, Canon 1, Fen 1, Tract. 1, Cap. 8.

[62]Followers of Thessalus, son of Hippocrates, physician to the court of Archelaus of Macedonia, putative author of some of the spurious books of Hippocrates.

[63]George Sarton, *Lilium Medicinae*. In *Medieval Studies in Honor of J. D. M. Ford*, V.T. Holmes and A. J. Denomy, eds. (Cambridge, Massachusetts, 1948), p. 239.

[64]Philagrius, a Greek physician in the second half of the 4th century A.D. who wrote a commentary on Hippocrates and a treatise on kidney stones; see J. F. K. Hecker, *Geschichte der Heilkunde*. (Berlin, 1829), p. 429.

cent.),[65] Guy Faba,[66] William of Saliceto (Guliemus de Placentia), Master Bertinus de Rabis of Parma,[67] Bruno Longoburgo (Brunus), Bernuncus of Parma[67], Serapion and Abucasis.

At the end of this potpourri, Leonard warns his students: "Trust incompletely anything cited by authority unless it can be explained by experiment or by reason." Much emphasis has been placed upon medieval subservience to tradition, yet we have here an example of a scholar cautioning against uncritical acceptance.

The author embarks on a classification of the agents causing head injury, and thereafter classifies wounds. The former appears in the Hippocratic corpus[68] and in medieval times as early as the Four Masters.[69] Medieval tradition clearly recognized the dangers of closed head injuries. Avicenna's[70] dictum, "Often the skull is injured and the skin uninvolved" was confirmed by Lisfranc,[71] Roger,[72] Bruno da Longobardo[73] and Guy de Chauliac.[74]

At the close of the fourth chapter, Leonard remarks: "At times the head is hit in one place and the bone itself fractures in another." This is almost, but not quite, the principle of *contra coup*. According to modern concept, a fracture or brain injury may occur directly opposite the site of impact. Leonard observes that the bone fracture may occur at a point distant to the site of impact. Egyptian sources[75] were first to make this observation and the Hippocratic school[76] and Celsus[77] likewise relate that the blow may be received in one part of the head and the fracture occur in another. Paul of

[65]Italian physician of the 14th century; see Alfred Chevelalier, *Répertoire des Sources Historique du Moyen Age*. (Paris, 1907), p. 1578.

[66]Guidonus Faba, Professor of Letters at Bologna during the 14th century? Unlikely.

[67]I am unable to identify Bernucus and Bertinus of Parma. The authorities of the Biblioteca Palatina of Parma were kind enough to search the names for me and reported that they, too, were unable to identify them.

[68]*On Injuries of the Head*, 7–11.

[69]Daremberg, ref. 39, Book 1, Ch. 1.

[70]Avicenna, Canon 4, Fen 5, Tract. 3, Cap. 1: Multotiens accidit ut findatur craneum et non findatur cutis imo apostematur.

[71]Lisfranc II.1, *op.cit.*, ref. 6.

[72]Karl Sudhoff, *Studien zur Geschichte der Medizin: Chirurgie im Mittelalter*, Band 11–12. The Surgery of Roger Frugardi of Salerno, chapter 1.

[73]Bruno da Longoburgo, *Cyrurgia Parva*, Book 1, Tract. 8, Cap. 4, in ref. 6.

[74]Guy de Chauliac, Tract. 3, Doc. 2, Cap. 1.

[75]James H. Breasted, *The Edwin Smith Surgical Papyrus*. (Chicago, 1930), p. 66.

[76]Hippocrates, *On Injuries of the Head*, 8: "A bone may be injured in a different part of the head from that in which the person has received the wound."

[77]Celsus, *De Medicina* VIII.4.7.

Aegina (fl. seventh century) seems most closely to approximate the modern concept: "The fissure is discovered which appears to them to have been occasioned by the blow on the opposite side."[78] This version seems to have been forgotten during the Middle Ages.[79]

Leonard advised his student that there is a point beyond which medical treatment is of no avail [71^v]. Such advice rests on firm medieval tradition. St. Gregory had previously criticized the practice of plying the incurable with medications.[80] In Leonard, one perceives a pervasive sincerity and humility, which the reader readily encounters in the text. Leonard's reverent regard for, and subservience to, the will of the Supreme Arbiter serves to underscore Thompson's remarks: "In his humanity towards his patients and his desire to do the utmost to help them, the medieval physician was equal to the best of our medical men today."[81]

In Chapter V, the author considers the general methods of evacuating excessive humors. Celsus[82] details the list: "substances are withdrawn by blood letting, cupping, purging, vomiting, rubbing. . . by body exercises of all kinds, by abstinence, by sweating." With regard to cupping, if the skin is cut before the cup is stuck, the cup extracts blood; if the skin is intact, wind.[83]

The importance of astrology [71^v] is discussed next, in relation to the patient's health. Leonard's observation, taken together with his *Judgments of the Revolution*, account for the scorn subsequently heaped upon him as a "miserable astrologer." In the early Middle Ages, astrology attracted scant interest and, until the twelfth century, "lived only in the form of academic discussion."[84] In a way,

---

[78]Paulus Aegineta, VI.90. Trans. Francis Adams, *The Seven Books of Paulus Aegineta*. (London, 1846), vol. 2, p. 432.

[79]Warren R. Dawson, *A Leechbook, or Collection of Medical Recipes of the Fifteenth Century*. (London, 1934), pp. 4, 843. Dawson stated that the principle of *contra coup* is found in his work, but I have not been able to confirm this.

[80]Sister Mary Emily Keenan, "St. Gregory of Nyssa and the Medical Profession." *Bull. Hist. Med. 15:*155, 1944.

[81]*Historiographical Essays in Honor of James Westfall Thompson,* J. L. Cote and E. N. Anderson, eds. (Chicago, 1938)

[82]Celsus, *De Medicina* II.9. I am aware that Celsus is supposed to have been rediscovered only at the close of Medieval times, but tenth to twelfth century MSS. were inventoried in Vatican, Paris and Florence libraries, and it seems to me that the substance of his ideas were known. See the review of Pearl Kibre, *The Library of Pico della Mirandola* (New York, 1936) in *Isis 26:*159--161, 1936.

[83]Celsus, *De Medicina* I.8.40.

[84]Theodore Otto Wedel, *Medieval Attitude toward Astrology*. (New Haven, 1920), p. 67.

the ignorance of astrology paralleled the unfamiliarity with ancient medical texts. Knowledge was limited to a handful of manuscripts, often corrupted by scribal transcription, a few magic texts, antidotaries,[85] etc. With the appearance of the great translations of Constantine the African in the eleventh century and the Toledo translations of the twelfth century, the dazzling range of Greek and Arabic science, of which astrology is venerable part, reached the western notice. Albertus, Peter of Abano and Arnold of Villanova were all enthralled with the new subject.[86] The Four Masters[87] declare that just as the moon is the origin of the humors of the earth, the humors of the brain react to lunar phases. Roger[88] also notes this affinity. Bernard of Gordon[89] describes the effects of each quarter in an elaborate and ingenious schema. No learned physician after the fourteenth century could fail to refer to astrology in connection with the health of his patient.

The author speaks [71^v] of repletion. This is defined by Galen,[90] citing Hippocrates, as an "abundance of humidity." Thereafter, Leonard interjects yet another case of brain injury, this concerning a peasant who survived a wound of the gray matter and who "is at present healthy."

Leonard begins his discussion of the therapeutic regime [71^v]. The necessity for a large room with good ventilation is stressed. Soranus[91] instructs the physician to "have the patient lie in a moderately light and warm room." Bernard of Gordon,[92] on the other hand, argues for a large room but proposes that the windows be kept closed. This disagreement in hygiene between the merits of the open-and-shut window persists down to the present. Concerning room temperature, Galen[93] states that cold is the ultimate

---

[85]Corner, ref. 58, p. 10.

[86]David Eugene Smith, "Medicine and Mathematics in the Sixteenth Century." *Ann. Med. Hist. 1:*125, 1917.

[87]Daremberg, ref. 39, Book 1, ch. 1: Et luna est mater humiditatis terrę nascentum et tunc humiditas cerebri augitur et ebulit cerebrum cum intus in magna quantitate humiditas eius nequeat contineri.

[88]I. Reichborn-Kjennerud, "The School of Salerno and Surgery in the North during the Saga Age." *Ann. Med. Hist. 9:*321, 1937.

[89]William G. Lennox, "Bernard of Gordon on Epilepsy." *Ann. Med. Hist. N.S. 3:*373, 1941.

[90]Galen, *De Locis Affectis* III.8.

[91]I. E. Drabkin, "Soranus and his System of Medicine." *Bull. Hist. Med. 25:*510, 1951.

[92]Lennox, ref. 89.

[93]Galen, *De Usu Partium* VIII.2.

harm. Leonard recommends fowl for the diet, as did the Four Masters[94] earlier. Examination of the pulse is recommended; Galen was intrigued by the pulse and wrote extensively on the subject.[95] Avicenna, too, saw in the pulse a close reflection of the illness. Urinalysis is also commended as an important aid to the diagnosis, following the suggestion of Hippocrates in the *Prognostics*.[96] Bed rest and supportive treatment are detailed. Sleep is important. Lisfranc,[97] however, cautions against excessive slumber which enfeebles the virtues, whereas insufficient sleep sharpens the humors. In general, a proper balance was more commonly recommended, in conformity with the sentiments of the Hippocratic physicians[98] who advised: "As regards sleep, the patient should follow his usual habits and spend the day awake and the night asleep."

In circumstances where the wound has not an open passageway to permit discharge, and to allow the brain to expire, Leonard recommends the use of his *moicula* [72^{r}]. What is this instrument? It would appear at this point that the instrument has something to do with incising bone. Later in the chapter, however, Leonard furnishes additional description when he states, "at which time or thereabouts the physician attempts to remove the bone of the skull, and this with a moicula."

The *moicula* appears to be unique to Leonard. The instruments in common use during medieval times were described by Guy de Chauliac,[99] whose descriptions are difficult to improve upon (Fig. 1).

There are six principal instruments and one should have three large, small, and medium sizes of each:

1. Trepans are used to make holes to raise the bone—Galen makes them like terebelli with a projecting ring a little above the cutting point of the trepan so that, when perforating the bone, it will not fall on the dura mater (A). The Parisians, in

---

[94]Daremberg, ref. 39, Book 1, ch. 1.

[95]Libellus de Pulsibus ad Tirones; Libri quatuor de Pulsuum Differentiis; Libri quatuor de Pulsibus Diagnoscendis; Libri quatuor de Causis Pulsuum; Libri quatuor de Praesagitione ex Pulsibus; Synopsis Sexdecim Librorum de Pulsibus; Pulsuum Compendium.

[96]*Prognostics*, 12.

[97]Tract. 1, Cap. 2.

[98]*Prognostics* 10.

[99]Guy de Chauliac, Tract. 3, Doc. 2, Cap. 1: Instrumenta capitalis sunt sex. . . Also, W. A. Brennan, *Guy de Chauliac.* (Chicago, 1923), p. 96.

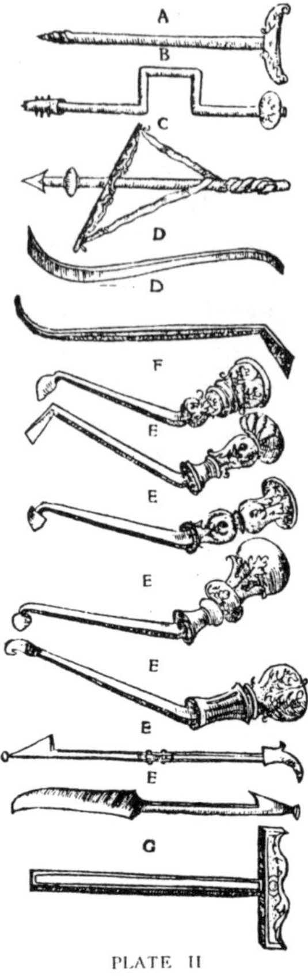

Figure 1. *Instruments of Guy de Chauliac. (Guy de Chauliac,* On Wounds and Fractures *[1363], Tract. III, Dec. 2, Cap. 1. Illustration taken from translation by William Brenna, [1923], p. 96, who composited the illustrations from the printed texts, e.g, Simon Rigaud, [Lyon, 1542].)*

order to reduce the number suitable for different operations, pierce the trepans with holes above the point and insert pegs (B). The Bolognese make them in the shape of a lance so that the acute part can enter, but the wider part is prevented from entering inadvertently (C).

2. Separators connect one perforation to the other and they are of two kinds: the first is French; the second is Bolognese, curved, and with the end one can make an elevator.
3. Elevators to raise the trepanned bone and separate it (D).

4. Rugines enlarge the incision and are of the form of the rugines of carpenters (E).
5. Lancets smooth and remove by means of a lenticular in the form of a lentil which it has for a head and on account account of the split lenticular shape at its point (F).
6. The mallet strikes the lancet from the end. It ought be of a heavy material, weighing much for a small mass and then also its sound is dulled (G).

Leonard alludes to the trepans in common practice and uses the terms trepan perforator (which corresponds to the terebelli) and the iron trepan (which probably corresponds to either the Parisian or Bolognese trepan—probably the latter). With these instruments, a hole is bored around the depressed fracture. The fracture can be then lifted up with an elevator, or a hole bored in bone and the hole enlarged with a rugine. The iron instrument can be heated to coagulate the blood vessels (*trepano ferrino*).

But where does the *moicula* fit into this scheme? Two new instruments appeared during the Renaissance. One, the crown trepan, was thought to have been rediscovered by de Carpi.[100] The second, a peculiar corkscrew instrument resembles the contemporary Italian corkscrew. The latter appears in German Renaissance texts, the former in Italian works of the sixteenth century.

Now, in Chapter V.2 of the 5th Tractate on *Osteology*, Leonard begins by declaring: "The saws with which we have to cut bone ought to be of diverse manner. . . There is the round saw perforating in the manner of a terebelus, such as the trepan. There is also a round saw with a ducal form with teeth around it. . ."[101]

The latter, the ducal form with teeth, appears to be the crown trephine (*modiolus*) later described by sixteenth century surgeons. It would seem that the crown trephine was unknown to early

---

[100]Edouard Nicaise, *La Grand Chirurgie de Guy de Chauliac*. (Paris, 1890), p. 268. In the illustrations of the sixteenth century, the instrument is called the "Modiolus, or Ancient Trephine." See J. S. Milne, *Surgical Instruments in Greek and Roman Times*. (Oxford, 1907), pp. 131--133.

[101]*De Ossibus*, Tract. 5, Cap. 2: Serre cum quibus secare debemus ossa debent esse diversarum manerierum et hoc propter necessitatem ut non affenatur hora sectionis membrum vicinum. Quedam est serra rotunde perforens in modum terebelli sicut sunt trepani. Quedam est alia serra rotunda ad gamant sunt cum dentibus ad intra nunc ad extra. Quedam est serra que dicunt raspa nunc reda nunc aliqualiter plicata ut levatorium nunc curva ad formam novitunum et iste raspe sunt cum dentibus sicut sunt lune.

medieval surgeons. Paul of Aegina mentions that it was not used in his day and that only the trepan was employed.[102]

No mention of the crown trephine is found in the list of instruments cited by Guy de Chauliac, nor in the works of the earlier surgeons.[103] The new instrument mentioned by Leonard is called the *moicula*. Now the crown trepan was known to the ancients as the *modiolus*. It is quite possible that *moicula*[104] is some corruption of the word *mochlia*, used by Galen to mean the "reduction of bone from an unnatural place." If so, Malgaigne is correct in crediting Leonard with the reintroduction of the crown trephine, mentioned in the section on Osteology, and I suggest that this is the *moicula* mentioned in *De Fractura Cranii*. I further conjecture that the instrument possibly had been in use for general bone surgery (Leonard mentioned it under general bone instruments) and that Leonard adopted it for use on the skull.

Leonard uses albumen [72r] to arrest scalp bleeding. Of course, other methods were known: medications, ligatures, cautery, or "the blood's own nature," as the Four Masters[105] refer to intrinsic clotting properties. Although not mentioned in the *De Fractura Cranii* or the *De Nervis*, the transfixation of the blood vessel was described elsewhere by Leonard and remains to this day an important aid to hemostasis. When tying off blood vessels, the surgeon finds that ligatures sometimes slip off, resulting in rebleeding. What Leonard did was pass the needle through the wall of the blood vessel before tying it, so that the ligature cannot slip. This is recounted in the following passage: ". . . and afterward tie that [vessel] with a linen tie, and, that it better hold, stitch that vein with the point of the needle and, with the tie, pass it around the vessel. . ."[106] Pain is to be avoided at all costs since, according to Galen, it is a cause of attracting matter to the wounded area and of engendering suppuration." This Guy de Chauliac[107] confirms. Leonard [72r] advises that the hair be shaved before the wound is treated. This practice also appears in the Salerno student's notebook,[108] and in the works

[102]Paulus Aegineta, VI.90.

[103]Karl Sudhoff, *Studien zur Geschichte der Medizin: Chirurgie im Mittelalter*, 2nd part. (Leipzig, 1918), Band 11--12, pp. 6, 87.

[104]Bartholomaeus Castelli, *Lexicon Medicum*. (Nuremberg, 1682), s.v.

[105]Daremberg, ref. 39, Book 1, ch. 1.

[106]See introductory material on the life of Leonard of Bertapaglia.

[107]Guy de Chauliac, Tract. 3, Doc. 2, Cap. 1.

[108]Henry E. Sigerist, "A Salernitan Student's Surgical Notebook," *Bull. Hist. Med. 14:*505, 1943.

of Bruno da Longoborgo[109] and Lisfranc.[110] Digestives [72ᵛ] have a place in the treatment of certain skull fractures. A digestive is a substance that assuages pain and defines necrotic tissue.[111] In this connection, Leonard reproves the practice of the barbers, who reach for the knife before trying nonsurgical methods. At times, he says, the digestives do their work so well that trepanation is not required. Doubtless what he had in mind are the small loose or detached fragments which digestives might be able to liquefy.

In the discussion of wound healing, Leonard appears to be dealing with second intention [73ʳ]. As we understand it today, second intention occurs when wound edges do not heal directly, but only after granulation tissue fills in the gap. Guy de Chauliac states,[112] "When the divided parts are reunited by the medium of some foreign substances. . . this medium is called the porus sarcoides (granulation tissue) and is made of a grosser humor than for the flesh." Over the wound, Leonard recommends the placement of a cupping bowl [73ʳ]. Brass and glass bowls had earlier been employed, but by the fifteenth century glass predominated. Leonard used the cupping glass to prevent the dressing from impinging on the brain. This appears to be an original suggestion, anticipating the plaster of Paris coverings used in Cushing's day. The Four Masters,[94] mindful of the danger of pressure, recommended light dressings.

Leonard cites another case of vexing posttraumatic seizure [73ᵛ]. The medieval physician, following Galen,[113] regarded seizures as having three modes of origin. First, seizures could result from intrinsic brain disease (idiopathic) or from the head injury, as the Hippocratic physicians first suggested. In this connection, Galen held that such seizures resulted from a plethora of brain humors which occluded the ventricles, especially the middle (third) and posterior (fourth). Second, seizures could be caused by a sympathetic reflex of humors to the brain as a result of heart disease or abundance of bile. Third, seizures could be caused by the brain's sympathetic response to disease originating in certain other parts

---

[109]Bruno da Longoburgo, Book 1, Cap. 8: *De Extractione Telorum et Astellarum*, Cap. 4.

[110]Lisfranc, II.1.

[111]Joannes de Vigo, *Practica in Chirurgia*. (Lyon, 1561) Book 3, Tract. 1, Cap. 7.

[112]Guy de Chauliac, Tract. 3, Doc. 1, Cap. 1.

[113]Owsei Temkin, *The Falling Sickness*. (Baltimore, 1945), pp. 61--129.

of the body. Such might occur, for example, when a seizure begins in the limb and slowly ascends to the brain. Galen likened the phenomenon to the upward sweep of poison following a scorpion bite. Thus Galen teaches that, if a convulsion occurs in a limb, the cause must be sought in the peripheral nerve which innervates the limb. Similarly, if the entire body convulses and the brain does not lose consciousness, the cause must be in the cervical cord. Accordingly, Leonard proposes that clonus be treated by bandaging or by rubbing the limb, and Bernard of Gordon[114] concurs.

Leonard alludes to the stages of illness: incipient, augmentation, establishment and decline [73^{v}]. This venerable classification persisted up to recent times, but lost its popularity with the waning of the infectious diseases. The author [73^{v}] alludes to head bandaging. Medieval physicians were extremely adept at bandaging, probably better than physicians today. Galen[115] has a separate chapter on the subject and recounts 70 methods. Leonard [74^{r}] begins with a description of the remedies required for the treatment of head injuries. He is anxious to expose the student to every modality which, as a practicing surgeon, he has found of value. Barley gruel is recommended, and had enjoyed great popularity since the Hippocratic recipes.[116] He cites several "experiments" [74^{v}]. An experiment is a remedy to be tried. If it works, the diagnosis is confirmed. In modern parlance, we call this a "therapeutic test." Leonard cautions against the use of wild fowl from the marshes [75^{v}]. This warning had also been sounded by Celsus,[117] Bernard of Gordon,[118] John of Gaddesden, and Jacme d'Argramont.[119] Wine is also to be avoided, he tells us, and if used (Jacme d'Argramont)[119] it should be watered.

The author has a unique section commencing on [76^{r}] devoted to diagnosis of skull fractures. Among the earlier methods, Galen[120] lists history, inspection, and palpation. Leonard searches for the site where humors rise when the patient exhales, where raucous noises are heard when the skull is percussed ("cracked pot sign"),

[114] Lennox, ref. 89.

[115] Galen, *De Fasciis*.

[116] *Regimen in Acute Diseases* 4.

[117] Celsus, *De Medicina* II.21--24.

[118] Lennox, ref. 89, pp. 273, 300.

[119] C.-E. A. Winslow and M. L. Duran-Reynals, "Jacme d'Agramont and the First of the Plague Tractates." *Bull. Hist. Med. 22:*747--765, 1948.

[120] Guy de Chauliac, Tract. 3, Doc. 2, Cap. 1.

and where pain is felt when a knife held between the patient's teeth is plucked. He inspects the wound to see what happens when medication has been put into it. Hippocrates[121] mentions the practice of having the patient chew on a stalk of fennel. Guido and Peter de Argelata place a straw between the patient's teeth and pluck on a cord.[122] Bruno[123] uses palpation. Galen[124] proposes the patient blow on a trumpet to determine whether the submeningeal space fills with air. Roger[125] uses palpation, as do the Four Masters.[126] The latter also cite the merits of having the patient exhale with closed nostrils and mouth. In general, Leonard's diagnostic tests [75^{v}-76^{v}] closely resemble those used by his predecessors. He stresses that the inner table of the skull can be fractured although the outer table is intact. For the medieval surgeon, this had a compelling importance, since he had no direct way to determine conclusively whether or not the inner table pressed on the brain.

Palpation notwithstanding, if symptoms and clinical findings support the diagnosis of intracranial pressure, the surgeon was obliged to decompress. Note mention of the diploë [76^{v}], which nourish the brain. This is discussed in greater detail by Galen[127] and the Four Masters.[128]

In his eleventh sign, Leonard advocated the insertion of a wick as a diagnostic aid to establish skull fracture. This, too, is a form of experiment, although not referred to as such. Theodoric[129] also recommends *ponas super fissuram encaustrum ut per illud fissure magis apareat manefeste*. If the discharge turns out to be *nigredo* (black discharge), then, Avicenna teaches,[130] the outlook is bleak.

Leonard demonstrates his ingenuity when discussing the cupping glass. As mentioned earlier, others had noted the harm caused by a tight dressing around the head after bone had been re-

[121] *Coan Prognostics* 28.

[122] Joannes de Vigo, *Practica in Chirurgia.* (Lyon, 1561) Book 3, Tract. 1, Cap. 4.

[123] Bruno da Longoburgo, *Cyrurgia Parva*, Book 1, Tract. 8, Cap. 4, ref. 6.

[124] Friederich Falk, *Galens Lehre von Gesunden und Kranken Nervensystem*. (Leipzig, 1871), p. 10.

[125] Sudhoff, ref. 103, "Surgery of Roger," I.5.

[126] Daremberg, ref. 39, Book 1, ch. 6.

[127] Galen, *De Usu Partium* IX.6; XVI.12.

[128] Daremberg, ref. 39, Book 1, ch. 6: Nota quod inter tabulas istas sunt vene et arterie que diferunt sanguinem ad craneum nutriendum.

[129] Theodoric, II.6.

[130] Avicenna, Canon 4, Fen 5, Tract. 3, Cap. 1.

moved.[131] But, if a cupping glass were to be placed above the wound before the dressing were applied, the brain would be protected. Furthermore, the glass gives a better contour to the dressing and permits discharges to escape from the wound. Leonard's recommendation that holes be placed in the glass corresponds to the perforated metal cranioplasties used in the recent past.

Leonard concludes with a list of the symptoms encountered in the first seven days following head injury [76v]. Note that pulse irregularity is mentioned, a feared sequel of intracranial pressure. The list resembles the symptoms and signs found in Guy de Chauliac,[132] but lacks his elegance.

---

[131]Daremberg, ref. 39, Book 1, ch. 2.

[132]Guy de Chauliac, Tract. 3, Doc. 2, Cap. 1: Pain, scotoma, vertigo, hot face, orificial bleeding, garbled speech, stupor, incontinence, vomiting, motor weakness.

V

Textual Criticism

The manuscript used in this study is found in the collection of the Riccardian Library in Florence (Fig. 1). Microfilms of the manuscript were obtained in 1950 and 1984. The manuscript, numbered 858 (new number), is of parchment and measures 205 mm. × 278 mm. It has 108 folia, newly numbered and gathered into nine sesternia. The first 82 folia have the old numbers. The handwriting is humanistic cursive. The manuscript consists of two parts; the first (folia 1--84), which concerns this study, was written by a single scribe and contains the *Chirurgia* and *Astrologia* of Leonard of Bertapaglia.

The incipit begins on 1*r*:[1] "We therefore begin in the Name of our Lord, Jesus Christ and His Mother, the glorious Virgin Mary, who inspires me and you and all wanderers in the byways of knowledge and the paths of truth and virtue, and reproves the bestial appetites and strengthens my heart. Here are the prescriptions given in the year of our Lord MCCC/XXI to his colleagues by Master Leonard of Bertapalia, who was delegated to lecture by the rectors of the reigning duke in the University of Padua on the 3rd, 4th and 5th fens (sententiae) of the 4th *Canon* of Avicenna. Here follows the chapter concerning pus."

The explicit[2] is found in 82*r* and begins: "Finished, therefore,

---

[1]Incipiamus ergo in nomine domini nostri Iesu Christi et gloriose virginis Marie eiusque matris qui me et vos omnes adiscentes confirmet et in via cognoscendi in semita veritatis et virtutis et reprimat appetitus bestiales et conroboret cor meum (1.14). Hac sunt recepte date per magistrum Leonardum de Bertapalia Anno domini M.CCCC/XXI suis sociis qui deputatus fuit ad lecturam per rectores ducali dominii in studio Paduano et hoc super tertiam et quartam et quintam senteniam 4[i] Canonis Avicenne. Sequitur capitullum de flegmone. . .

[2]Expl. C. 82[a], 1.17: Sit ergo gratia brevitatis nunc finis huic tractati de aspectibus compilatim et in hac forma abreviationes perductum per Leonardum de Bertapalia Peduanum Anno MCCCC.CXXIIII[0] de mense Martii. Deo gratias.

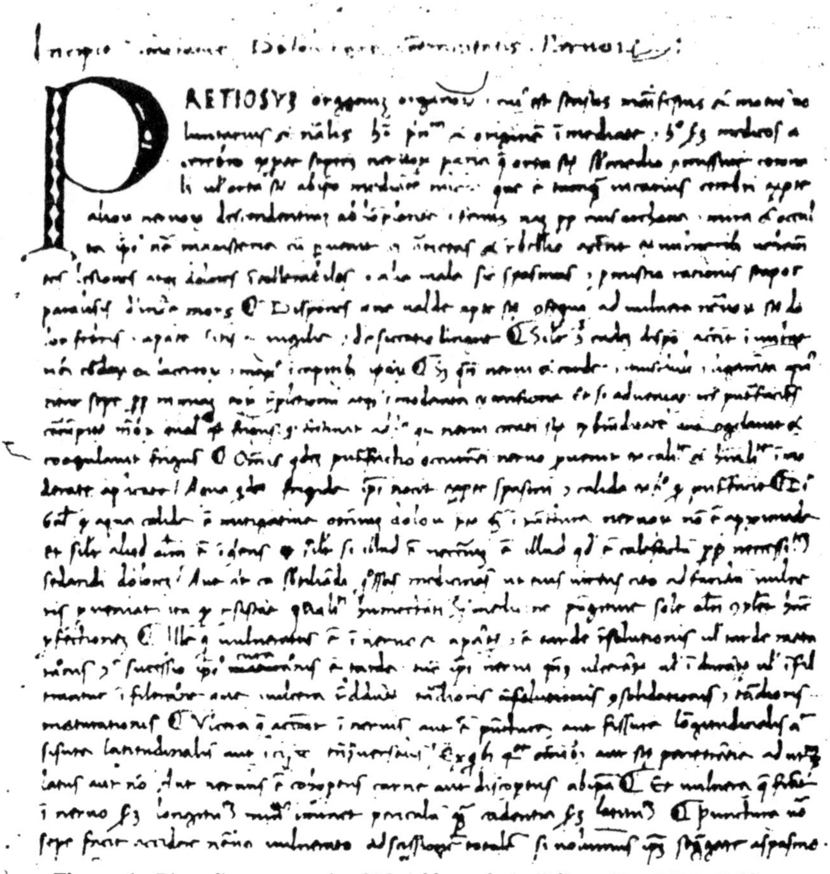

Figure 1. *Riccardian manuscript 858 (old number), Folium 61r, 1424. (Biblioteca Riccardiana, Florence, Italy).*

with thanks for its brevity, this tractate concerning related aspects, in this abbreviated form, produced by Leonard of Bertapalia, 1424 in the month of March. Thanks be to God."

This incipit differs slightly from those contained in other manuscripts studied by the late Lynn Thorndike. For those who seek a critical comparison of the various incipits, attention is directed to the masterful survey by Thorndike, whose exemplary scholarship leaves little to be added. Several manuscripts have found their way into the collections at the Laurentian Library at Florence, the Wolfenbuettel, Prague, National Library of Naples, the Bodleian Library,[3] and elsewhere.[4] These manuscripts are really copies of the lecturer's notes or, in substance, the lecture

itself. Custom called for the professor lecturer, be he the ordinary (morning) or extraordinary (afternoon) lecturer, to submit his course to the university stationers, who would make sufficient and accurate copies (exemplars)[5] for the use of the students enrolled in the course. These exemplars could be made by a single scribe (as in our Riccardian manuscript No. 858) or they could be divided into units of four folia (*peciae*)[6] and the units "mass-produced" by several scribes, each assigned a single pecia. Ownership of a manuscript was prohibitively expensive for all but the most wealthy of students. The manuscript was arbitrarily divided into *punctae*, which the lecturer was required to reach in his lecture. If he failed to do so, he could be reported to the rector by denunciators and fined.

From the standpoint of grammar and composition, the work of Leonard must be judged by standards differing from other surgical works of the Middle Ages. In particular, two important differences seem apparent. First, the surgeries of Theodoric, Guy de Chauliac, and others were conceived as complete surgical works. Leonard, however, was specifically charged and required to present to the university stationer only a commentary to the 4th *Canon* of Avicenna, so that the range of his enterprise was limited. Had he intended to write a complete surgical treatise, he would perhaps have elected to follow a different plan free from academic strictures. Second, the grammar of Leonard is crude,[7] even by medieval standards. Leonard seems to have collected contemporary criticism on this very point. "Let no one accuse me of coarse speech, since I have said many things complicated by obscurity and confusion,"[8] he retorts. However, if we examine the text carefully, there are

---

[3]Lynn Thorndike, "Another Manuscript of Leonard of Bertipaglia and John de Tracia." *Bull. Inst. Hist. Med. 4:*257, 1936.

[4]Karl Sudhoff, *Studien zur Feschichte der Medizin,* 11--12 (Leipzig, 1918), p. 509, reports a MS., probably an abstract made by a student, called *Dicta Leonhardi (de Bertapalia) in Chirurgia.*

[5]Hastings Rashdall, *Universities of Europe in the Middle Ages*. (Oxford, 1895), vol. 1, p. 191.

[6]For controls of *peciae* by the *peciarii*, see Lynn Thorndike, *University Records and Life in the Middle Ages*. (New York, 1944), p. 166.

[7]Antoine Portal, *Histoire de l'Anatomie et de la Chirurgie*. (Paris, 1770), vol. 1, p. 238: 'Son language est dur et barbare."

[8]Nemo michi crimen imponat et prolixitate rudis sermonis cum multa complicata obscuritate et confusione dixerim. Cod. Biscon. 13, f. 27^{v}; Cod. Sloane 3863, fol 51, quoted from Thorndike, "The Manuscript Text of Cyrurgia of Leonard of Bertipaglia." *Isis 1:*266, 1926.

unmistakable evidences that we are reading the spoken language. Not only was the lecturer required to make his point, but he had to express himself in a manner capable of holding the student's attention. Surely it was no easy task to lecture in a small, stuffy room filled with foul-smelling, itching, boisterous medical students. Adding to the lecturer's woes, many students came from distant reaches to the compass, each with a varying command of late medieval academic Latin, notwithstanding the enrollment requirements at a time when even vernacular pronunciation changed every thirty miles. Thus, despite the criticism of Leonard by his colleagues, we may presume that his simple, straightforward medieval Latin must have evoked the gratitude of his students.

Why did a lecture course survive 500 years in many widely dispersed manuscripts? A posteriori, one might suspect that the popularity of the lecturer with his students compelled the stationers to make many exemplars. We may further presume that his contemporaries or his students, if not his patients, held Leonard in unusually high esteem. Concerning the wide dispersal of manuscripts, one need but recall the words of Thompson:[9] "Books, like men, have their fates. Some meet solitary and tragic ends; some fall in holocausts; and some, after strange vicissitudes, narrow escapes, and long wanderings, find peaceful asylums where, nursing their scars and mellowed by experience, they will relate something of their adventures to the curious."

For the incunabula, I have used the edition of 1498, available to me through the kindness of the librarians of the Rare Book Room of the New York Academy of Medicine. The incunabular edition is an anthology containing the works of many other distinguished medieval physicians. Leonard was chosen to represent fifteenth century surgeons.

Several editions are said[10] to have preceded the 1498 edition. This assertion was critically analyzed by Thorndike[11] who was somewhat skeptical. "Of the editions of 1490 and 1497, I have

---

[9]James W. Thompson, *The Medieval Library*. (New York and London, 1965), p. 647.

[10]See Edouard Nicaise, *La Grande Chirurgie de Guy de Chauliac*. (Paris, 1890), p. cxxix, who quotes Brunet, stating that the printer of 1498, Bonetus Locatellus, published in 1490 a less complete edition. I think that he refers to the edition of 1497 (Octavianus Scotus).

[11]Lynn Thorndike, *Science and Thought in the Fifteenth Century*. (New York and London, 1963), pp. 62--63.

found little trace. . . they are not. . . recorded in Hain's *Repertorium Bibliographicum*[12] and its various supplements or in any other catalogue of incunabula that I have seen." I have reexamined Hain and have found an edition of 1490 printed by Octavianus Scotus, containing the surgery of Guy de Chauliac. Further, Hain lists an edition of 1497 which was an anthology containing the surgery of Guy de Chauliac as well as the other authors appearing in the subsequent editions. The publisher in both cases was Octavianus Scotus. Thus, the integrity of the publisher's assertion is born out and the surmise of Elroy,[13] who postulated an earlier condensed edition of 1490, is confirmed.

The incunabular edition of 1498 (Fig. 2) contains the *Cyrurgia* of Guy de Chauliac, as well as the surgeries of Bruno, Theodoric, Roland, Lanfranc, Roger, and Bertapaglia. The work of Leonard begins on folio 233 (newly numbered 234) and concludes on 267 (newly numbered 265). The incipit begins on 233:[14] "Here are the reflections (*recollectio*) concerning the 4th Canon of Avicenna collected by the famous and singular doctor master Leonard Bertapalia and herein are wondrous secrets privy to him and me." The "me" problably refers to the editor. An alternative explanation would assign authorship to the scribe of the manuscript on which the printed edition was based.

The colophon[15] on folio 233 (old number) begins: "Here end the reflections of the famous doctor master Leonard Bertapaglia concerning the 4th Canon of Avicinne. The edition was arranged and financed by the nobleman Director Octavianus Scotus from the city of Monza. The overseer and art controller was Bonetus Locatellus of Bergamo. In the year of the Birth of the Healing Virgin 1498 on the 11th Kallendar of December (November 21)."

The large folio measures 310 mm. × 210 mm. and has black

---

[12]L. F. T. Hain, *Repertorium Bibliographicum*, vol. 2, p. 82.

[13]N. F. J. Eloy, *Dictionnaire Historique de la Médecine*. (Liege and Frankfort, 1755), vol. 1, p. 150.

[14]He sunt recollecte habit super quarto Avicenne ab egregro et singulare doctore magistro Leonardo Bertapalia et ibi sunt mirabile secreta habita ab eo et per me experta.

[15]Recollectarum egregi doctoris magistri Leonardi Bertapalie super quarto Cannonis Avicenne finis. Venetiis Impressarum mandato et expensis Nobilis Viri Domini Octaviani Scoti Civis Modestiensis cura et arte [the text reads *ante* but this appears to be a typographical error] Boneti Locatelli Bergomensis. Anno a salutifero virginali partii Millensimo quadrigentesimo nonagesimo octavo. Undecimo Kalendas Decembres.

lupinoꝝ.añ.ʒ.iiij.olei camomellini.olei sambucini.añ.ʒ.
iiij.pulueris lūbꝛicoꝝ.ʒ.ij.fiat empl'm.Sed oīa decoquā-
tur in lixiuio:ꝛ sic canonice opando oīs doloꝛ cessabit ꝛ lu
crabimini floꝛenū ꝛ honoꝛem.

Tractatus.IIII. De solutione cōtinui neruoꝛuꝫ.
De egritudinibus neruoꝝ spe
ctantib⁹ad cyrurgicū in vniuersali. CAP. I.

Preciosum oꝛganū oꝛganoꝝ in quo
est sensus manifestus:ꝛ
motus voluntarius ꝛ nālis:hꝫ pncipium ꝛ
oꝛiginē imediate:ꝛ hoc fm medicos:a cere-
bꝛo ex parte septem pariū neruoꝝ:que oꝛta
sūt a medio comissure coꝛonalis vł oꝛta sūt
ab ipso mediāte nuca:que est tanq̄ꝫ vicari⁹
cerebꝛi ex parte alioꝝ neruoꝝ descēdētiū ab hō plāta infe-
rius.Nam pter eius arcana ꝛ mira ꝛ occulta ipsius nature magisteria cū peuenerit ei ꝯtrietas accidūt ex vulneribus vehementes lesiones atqꝫ doloꝛes ꝛ intolerabiles:ꝛ
alia mala:sicut spasmus permixtio rōnis:stupoꝛ paralesis
deinde moꝛs.¶ Dispositiones que apte sunt consequi ad

Figure 2. *Leonard of Bertapaglia, Tractate IIII. (Reproduced from Recollectae super chirurgia IV canonis Avicennae,* [Venice, 1498], p. 256 [new number 255].)

letter type, two columns of 65 lines with woodcut ornamental capitals. Reference to the edition appears in Hain #4811, British Museum Catalogue #451, and Pellechet #3530.[16] The cover is reinforced parchment.

Venice was the publishing center of Europe at the close of the fifteenth century. It is said that almost two million volumes were printed in that city in the interval between the introduction of printing and 1500.[17] At least 100 printers plied their trade during the last decade, attracted by Venetian technology in paper production. Their products found a market not only in Venice and nearby Padua, but in the entire civilized world touched by very extensive Venetian commerce.

The idea for an anthology first occurred to Octavianus Scotus. As mentioned above, he had published the surgery of Guy de

---

[16] Marie Pellechet, *Catalogue général des Incunables*. (Paris, 1905), vol. 2, p. 451.
[17] John Clyde Oswald, *A History of Printing*. (New York, 1928), pp. 100--101.

Chauliac in 1490, which presumably had a satisfactory reception. In 1497, he first published the surgical anthology, the strong selling point, no doubt, being the work of Guy de Chauliac. It would be tempting to speculate that the anthology was tailored to the curriculum at Padua, but this assumption is hazardous since the *Cyrurgia* of Leonard was no longer prescribed reading. More likely, the collection was intended as a general reference, inasmuch as the scope of reading for medical students was no longer limited to the prescribed manuscripts. By 1498, publication of the anthology was turned over to the firm of Bonetus Locatellus. The latter was certainly no newcomer to medical publishing. The year before, he had published a work on Rases.[18] Possibly Octavianus Scotus had grown old—he had been publishing since at least 1483 (Augustine)[18] and had acquired distinguished titles of respectability. At any rate, Bonetus Locatellus appears tohave had a university connection. He specialized in the printing of learned Latin books and despised the vernacular.[19] As early as 1491, an arrangement was made between Bonetus Locatellus and Octavianus Scotus concerning publication of Burlaeus and Sacro Bosco,[20] so that the further arrangement for the transfer of publication rights of a surgical anthology was not extraordinary.

It may seem, on first reflection, that the chief expenses involved in publication of the manuscripts would be the costs of printing and paper. Actually, the largest expenses were the purchase of the manuscripts and their revision, collation, correction and preparation for typesetting.[21] Thus, major costs for the edition of 1498 had already been expended by Octavianus Scotus.

Bonetus Locatellus appears to have been a shrewd businessman. Engaged as he was in the publication of scholarly works, he took pains to protect his investments by securing a "privilege," or, as it is known today, a copyright. Thus, on April 19, 1497, it is recorded that he received no fewer than 14 privileges,[22] a very large number for that time. This, of course, did little to prevent

[18]Bernard Quaritch, *A Catalogue of Books Printed in Europe during the 15th and 16th Centuries*. (London, 1923), part 1, p. 54.

[19]Alfred W. Pollard, *Fine Books*. (New York, 1912), p. 69.

[20]Lathrop Harper, *A Selection of Incunabula*. (New York, 1930), p. 179.

[21]George H. Putnam, *Books and their Makers during the Middle Ages*. (New York, 1896), vol. 1, p. 412.

[22]Konrad Hackler, *A Study of Incunabula*, Tr. Lucy Osborn. (New York, 1933), p. 196.

determined pirating beyond the confines of Venice, but since the city was then the publishing center of Europe, the privilege probably was an effective restraint.

A comparison between the manuscript and the incunabular edition reveals at once evidence of extensive editing. In the incunabula's incipit, we encountered the expression concerning "secrets known to him and to me." Was the "me" a former student of Leonard's? If so, did he audit the lectures between 1420--26? Such seems unlikely, since seventy-odd years had elapsed from the time of the lectures to the edition of 1498. Leonard could have given his lectures later than 1426 (he died in Padua in 1463) and several versions of the manuscript may have circulated, edited by a student who worked in the stationer's. Nevertheless, the principal differences between manuscript and printed edition can most likely be attributed to editing at the time of the printed edition, i.e., 1497. Let the reader compare the printed and the manuscript versions and form his own conclusions.

For purposes of comparison, the two texts have been presented collectively. In particular, seven items of difference are apparent.

First, the incunabular grammar is more elegant. Consider the opening chapter of the *De Fractura Cranei*. The manuscript reads, *Primum notabilia fac que tu sis instructus in principis medicinae*. The incunabula reads, *Primum arbitror que oportet eus qui perfectus cyrurgicus esse cupit*. Disregarding the slight difference in meaning, one perceives the crudity and inelegance of the manuscript. But one must ever remember that the manuscript was *heard* while the incunabula was *read*. Moreover, the difference points up a deference to greater precision and changing standards. *Fractura capitis* in the manuscript became *fractura cranei* in the incunabula.

Second, the incunabular editor suppressed many of Leonard's boastful references. Tastes had altered in the elapsing decades of the fifteenth century, just as the tastes of today differ from those at the turn of our century. Leonard's self praise must have appalled the good editor. The manuscript states, "It is well that you study with the experienced physician (such as me) and see him operate different cases and awful illnesses. . .", the editor very properly omitted the "such as me." Unfortunately, such interesting passages as the parchment operation [69^r] were deleted from the printed text for the very same reason, to spare the reader self-serving pomposity.

Third, there is a tendency to omit tapestries of medieval argument. For example, the manuscript often uses *oportet ut. . .Ratio*. The incunabula tires of this stilted style and substitutes *oportet ut. . .quia*.

Fourth, we see the appearance of incunabular rubrics. To be sure, the editor is at times careless or inconsequential in the numbering, but there is little doubt that his rubrics are meant to be helpful, if not incisive. *Capitulum primum* [69v] *de fractum capitis in formam consilii in que continentur undicum notabilia* in the manuscript becomes in the incunabula *Sequitur de fractura cranei. Capitulum V*.

Fifth, all personal references ("my son, Fabricius") in the printed work are deleted or changed to another form of address [71v]. Thus, *Tu filii* becomes *amice*.

Sixth, in the printed work, the editor often ignores numbered items or paragraphs appearing in the manuscript, suggesting a rebellion against the medieval form. As an example, the *octivum notabile* of the manuscript becomes *aliud notabile* in the printed text [70v].

Seventh, superlatives are deflated. *Unquentum valde optimum* becomes *valde bonum.* [74v] *Numus periculoseora* becomes *nimum periculosa* [61v]. Notwithstanding, the incunabular editor has his own dramatic style: *Frigidum vero est valde inimicum* becomes in the printed edition *Frigidum vero mors* [61v].

There is no useful purpose in burdening the reader with a list of omitted words, transposed sentences, grammatical or proofreading errors appearing in the manuscript or printed texts. Leonard certainly never had cause to anticipate, nor did he intend, that his lecture notes would survive him, no more than a professor of today would expect immortality from his xerographed notes. That Leonard has survived must attest to more than chance and if some of us, uncharitably, cannot altogether discern the reasons, let us at least not revenge our perplexities by carping on his imperfections.

VI

Pharmacopoeia

Abici[1]	fir; *Pinus abies;* Oil of Siberian Fir
Absinth	wormwood; *Artemisia absinthium*
Acatia[2]	acia; Acacia from which gum arabic was made
Acetum	vinegar
Acorus	gladiola root; *Acorus Calamus*
Aggregativis	hortense
Agresta	hortense
Agrippe[3,6]	agripa; an ointment (Galen)
Albumen	white of egg
Alembicum	liquid used by craftsmen to separate silver from gold
Aloe	leaves of *Aloe cicatrina*
Altee preparate	*Althaea officinalis,* marshmallow
Aluminis rochie	crude alum from village of Roche in Syria
Ambobus	ambobaja
Amygdela	fruit of *Amygdalus communis*
Ammoniac	gum residue of *Ferula Grevifolia*
A[r]murica	horseradish, *Armoracea rusticana*
Anelinus	indigo
Anetum[2] **graveoleno**	dill; *Anethum graveolens*

Anis	Anis; *Pimpinella anisim*
Animals	ass, badger, bear, cat, fox, frog, goose, horse, leper pig, lizard, vulture.
Apium	wild celery; *Apium graveolens*
Apostolorum[3,5,6]	an ointment of 12 ingredients. Same number as the Apostles.
Arabici	gum arabic
Aresi	areca tree beetlenut; *Acreca catechu*
Argonus	argon ointment
Arzica	rice
Aristologia[3]	birthwort; *Aristolohia clematitis*
Armoniacum	armoniac; gum resin from the ammoniac plant; *Dorema ammoniacum*
Arundinis	arundinacea
Assa	hot gum; *Assarum bacca*
Avellana	fruit of Hazel tree; *Corylus avellana*
Basilium ointment	pitch, resin, wax and fat
Balavstiarum	balaustia; flowers of *Punica granatum*
Balsaminum	aromatic balm made from genus *Myrovapermum*
Ben	ben; *Moringa aperta*
Bdellium	bdellium; Gum residue resembling myrrh, from shrubs of genus *Commiphora*
Berbena	pimpernell; *Berberis vulgaris;* Barberry
Betonica[3]	betony; *Stachys betonica*
Bolo armonico[9]	bole armeniac; an astringent earth
Boragins	borage; *Borago officinalis*
Butyra	butter
Caladista[1]	Galactites

Calamite	A reed-like plant
Calaminarus	Zinc oxide
Calamentus	Calaminth, a plant of the genus *Calaminta*
Calatus	senna
Calx	limestone
Calce	Alumen Indium (Avicenna)
Calcida	*Centaurea calcitrapa*
Calcitis	vitriol
Calcanthum	vitriol (Avicenna)
Calidicon	chalk
Calendule	marigold; *Calendula officinalis*
Calignis[5]	chalk; seed pilygonon; snakeweed
Camemdreum	Chamaedrys, Avicenna; *Chamaedrys foemina*
Camomelinus[3]	camomile; *Anthemis nobilis*
Canamunte	cinnamon; Faciolota; *Laurus cinnamomum*
Cannabis[3]	hemp; *Cannabis sativa*
Cardamomic	cardamomum[2]; fruit of East Indian herb, *Amomum cardamomum*
Carum carvi	caraway-plant; *Carum carvi*
Caseus	cheese
Castoreo	castorium
Cassia	senna, dried leaves of one of the species of Cassia; wild cinnamon
Caulis	cabbage
Centaurea minoris	lesser century
Cepa	onion; *Allium cepa*
Cera	wax
Cera alba	white wax

Cere citrine	yellow wax
Cere nove	fresh wax
Cere rube	red wax
Cere viridis	green wax
Ceratonia silqua	xylocaractum
Ceratum	ointment made with wax
Ciclamin	cyclamen; *Cyclamen europaeum*
Cicuta ebrilus	cicuta; hemlock
Cicinum oleum	castor oil; *Ricinus communis*
Cimini	anis; Palmberg; Cymenum
Cochiis[7]	chochium root
Conium	hemlock; C. maculatum
Colofonie[3]	colophony; residue of distillation of crude turpentine and water
Costinus[1,2,6]	costus root; *Costus arabicus*
Cotula	mayweed
Crocus	saffron; *Crocus sativus*
Crystilium	psylium; *Plantago psyllium*
Cucurbita	gourd; *Cucurbita pepo*
Cucumus	cucumus; cucumber; *Cucumus sativis*
Cuminum cummin	*Cummin cyminum*
Cuscute cuscute	*Cuscuta major; C. europae,* etc.
Cypressi roasarum	cyprus rose; *Cyprus sempervirens*
Dactylus	Date
Delfinum	*Delphinum staphisagria;* stavesacre
Diacatholicon	laxative electory
Dialtee	unguentum of Althaea

Diaquylo[2,3]	diachylon; a lead plaster
Diptami dittany	*Origanum dictamnus*
Dragantus	dragon wort; *Dracunulus vulgaris* (Arum dracunculus)
Ebenus	ebony sawdust; *Deospyrus ebenum*
Ebulus	sambucus; dwarf elder; *Sambucus ebulus*
Elena or Enule	Campane; elecampane; *Inula helenium*
Exula anabula[8]	Spurge; *Daphani aureola*
Euforbio	euphorbium; an acrid gum resin obtained from Eurphorbia resinifera
Faba	bean
Faloneria	Hungarian herb similar to mallows
Farrea	nubes
Felix	felix; felix a fern
Fenugrecus	fenugreek; *Trigonella foenumgraecum*
Ferment	leaven
Phili pendula	*Spiriroea filipandula*; dropwort
Filago	cudweed; *Filago germanicus*
Filigo pini	mixture of gumma pini and bdellium
Fufurus	bran
Fuscus	black ointment of Galen *De Compositione Medicamentorum*
Galbanum	Galbanum; aromatic gum residue from juice of *Ferula galbaniflua*
Gala	Gallium; *Gallium luteum*
Galeopsis	*Galeopsis tetrahit*; hemp-nettle
Garlange[7]	galega

Gariofolorum	cloves; the dried flower bud of *Caryophyllus aromaticus*
Gentian	gentian; *Gentiana lutea*
Granatus	granate tree; *Punica granatum*
Pomgranate	fruit of the tree, rinds of the fruit
Gumma ara	gum araby from the plants of the genus *Acacia*
Gumma elemi	gum of myrrh
Gypsum, gipsum	gypsum
Gratia dei	a plaster for cleaning and healing wounds.
Hydra ivy	hedera; *Hedera helix*
Hypoquistidos	Longuedoc sap
Ireos	iris; *Iris germanica*
Junipus[3]	juniper; *Juniperus communis*
Lactuca	lettuce; *Lactuca sativa* cultivated or *L. sariola* wild
Lapis ematitis	blood stone; *Lapis haematites;* red oxide of iron
Lapis magnetus	magnetic rock
Lapis molaris	a stone which is heated and vinegar poured over it (Avicenna)
Lardona	lard
Laudanus, laudanum	Tincture of opium
Laurinus, laurus	laurel; *L. nobilis;* Laurel oil is made from berries
Laurus nobilis	bacca lauri; *Laurus nobilis*
Lepidum sativum	nasturcium; Cress; sulfurated volatile oil
Lentis orobi	lentils
Lens	*Lenticula patustria;* Avicenna

Lignus	meal made from the cockle; *Lychiis githago*
Lilia	Lily
Linum	flax; a plant of the genus *Linum* esp L. *usitatissimum*, a cultivated flax
Lithargo	litharge; a compound of red lead
Lixivum	a liquid containing dissolved potash
Lolium[3]	darnel; *Lolium temulentum*
Lotus	lotus
Lumba	worms
Lupinus	lupine; "touch me not"; *Lupinus albus*
Lupulus	hop plant; *Humulus lupulus*
Maiorana	majory
Malaviscus	wild mallows; *Malva sylvestris*
Marchasite	marchasitum; a stone
Marchantia	liverwort; *M. polymorpha*
Marciatonis[3]	marciaton ointment for joints; agrippe, diacylon, diatar-ascos, catholicon
Masticus	mastix; resin of the mastix tree *Pistacia lentiscus* (terpentine lentiscus)
Matris silve[5]	matrissylva; honeysuckle; *Asperula odorata*
Mater sylva	Core of wood
Mauve	malva; mallows; *Malva rotundifola* or *M. sylvestris*
Medulla	crurium asini; marrow of ass's leg
Melica	melissa; *Melissa officinalis*
Melle	honey
Melle apium	bee's honey
Melle rossa	rose honey

Mellilotum	melilot; melilot; *Melilotus officinalis*
Melo	melo; *Cucumus celo*
Menta	wild mint; *Mentha sylvestria et piperita*
Milefolium	yarrow
Milium	milium
Minimum	red lead
Mirasolis	sunflower
Marcasite	bismuth
Mirtinus	myrthe; *Myrta communis*
Mirre myrrh[3]	a gum residue from the tree *Commiphora abyssinica*
Mitigitivus[3]	a soothing remedy
Molenchini[1]	marble stone; lapus molochites
Molendinus	flying seeds
Molybdena	lead rock
Mumie	mumie; a liquid material said to be found in sepulcres, but, in fact, of extremely variable composition.
Nardinus[3]	nardine; spice; *Nardostachys jutamansi*
Nigelle	nigella; *Nigella sativa*
Nux muscanta	King nut; *Migristica moschata*
Oleagina	olive oil derivative
Oleum communis	common oil
Oleum lartericum	brick oil
Oleo olivo	olive oil
Oleo petrolei	mountain oil
Oleo roso	rose oil and oil, obtained from a mixture of rose petals and olive oil which has been heated gently, strained, and allowed to stand for several weeks

Olibanum	Olibanum, frankincense; a fragrant gum resin from trees of Genus *Boswellia*
Opoponaco	opopanax; a gum resin obtained from the roots of *Opoponax chironium* (Hercules' allheal)
Ordei	barley
Origanum	pennyroyal; *Mentha pulegium*
Orobus	gum lac; produced by a scale insect
Orobus	orobus; *Ervum ervilia*
Ova vitella	yolk of egg
Oxicrocus	oxicrocus[6]; saffron, dates, egg, tallow, etc. heated in fire
Pano albissima	very white bread
Pellepode	polypody; fern *Polypodium vulgare*
Peonia	peony
Peregrina	Rubia peregrina; wild madder
Perpole[1]	storax; Propolus
Persicorum	heart wort
Pimpernelle	pimpernel; *Pimpinella anisum*
Pinus	pine; *Pinus pinea*
Pinea	fruit of the above
Piper	pepper from nearly ripe berries of *Piper nigrum*
Piretrum	pellitory of Spain; *Anacyclus pyrethrum*
Pyretrum[2]	Chamomile; *Anthemis pyrethrum*
Pix alba	white pitch from *Pinus abies*
Pix navalis	pitch residue from distillation of Pix Liquida
Populeon[6]	an ointment from poplar leaves
Prasium[5]	leek; Marrubium
Primula veris[3]	Primrose; *Primula veris*

Propolis[1]	styrax
Pulegii[3]	pennyroyal from *Menta pulegium*
Pumice	pumice
Purtulaca	portulace; *Portulaca oleracea*
Rosa	rose
Rosa rubra	*Rosa gallica*
Rosa marina	rosemary; *Rosmarinus officinalis*
Rasini pini	resin of pine
Rutin	rutin; *Ruta graveolens*
Sal	salt
Sal gemme	sal gemmae; rock salt
Sal baurachiis	salt peter
Salvie	sage; *Salvia officinalis*
Sambucinus elder	*Sambucus nigra (Sambucuc ebulus)*
Sandra	sanguis draconis; dragon blood; a gum resin of *Dracaena draco* and other shrubs
Sanguinis	humani; human blood
Santolinus	wormwood (absinth)
Sarcocole, sarcocolla[6]	a gum from Persia
Savinus	oil from ravin tree
Scamonea	scamonea; *Convolvulus scammonia*
Scorie	plumbi; slag
Serapinum	serapinum; gum residue of *Ferula persica*
Serpilium	serpilium; wild thyme; *Thymus serphyllum*
Siligins	ferment; poorly defined
Sinaps	mustard; *Sinaps nigra* and *S. alba*
Sponga	sponge; *Lapis spongiae*; sponge calcium

Spuma	maris; pumex
Sulfur	sulfur
Sulfurus triti	trisulfate of arsenic
Sticados arabici	lavender; *Lavandula stoechas*
Storax	storax; a liquid resin from *Styrax officinalis*, solid storax called *Storax calamite*
Terpentina	terpentine; a residue from the terbinth tree *Pistacia terebinthus* or the oleoresin from other coniferous trees
Terra sigillata	Jerusalem soil
Thus olibanus	resin of the frankencense tree
Titymalus	titymalus; *Luphorbia verrucosa*
Trifolium	trefoil; *Trifolium fragiferum*
Tricitum africana	couch grass
Vicius	vetch; a plant of the genus *Vicia*
Vernix	vernix; a liquid resin
Vin	vinum; wine
Viscus quercinus	mistletoe
Ungarica	Hungarian herb also called faloneria, similar to mallow
Yspoi hyssop	*Hyssopus officinalis*
Zinziber	ginger; *Zingiber officinalis*

Footnotes

[1]Johan Jacob Woyt, *Gazophylacium*. (Leipzig, 1722)

[2]Celsus, *De Medicina*, Trans. W. G. Spenser. (London and Cambridge, Massachusetts, 1938), vol. 2, pp. xv-lxiii.

[3]Margaret Sinclair Ogden, *The Liber de Diversis Medicinis*. (London, 1938)

[4]Jacopo Dondi dall' Orologio, *Enumeratio Remediorum Simplicium et Compositorum ad affectus fere omnes*. Conrad Gessner, ed. *De Chirurgia Scriptores optimi quique veteres et recentiores*. (Zurich, 1555)

[5]Stephen Blancard, *Lexicon Medicum*. (Magdeburg, 1748)

[6]Warren R. Dawson, *A Leechbook, or Collection of Medical Recipes of the Fifteenth Century*. (London, 1934)

[7]Karl Sudhoff, *Studien zur Geschichte der Medizin,* vol. 13. Studien u. Text zur Fruemittelelterischen Rezeptliteratur. (Leipzig, 1923)

[8]Simon Paulli, *Flora Danica*. (Copenhagen, 1648)

[9]D'Arcy Power, *De Arte Phisicali et de Chirurgica of Master John Arderne, Surgeon of Newark*. (London, 1922), p. 21.

Index

Albucasis, xxii, 69, 118
Aesculapius, 69, 117
Albertus Magnus, 69, 117
Alexandria, xvi–xvii, 42, 51
Alexandrian School, 43
Anaxagoras, 69, 117
Anesthesia, denervation, 3, 35, 37
Animal spirit, 117
Apoplexy, 59
Aristotle, 43
Arnold of Villanova, 47, 115, 117, 120
Arosboth, 114
Artery, superficial temporal, 114
Astrology, 119–120
Avicenna, ix, xvii, 7, 29, 35, 37, 43–49, 55, 57, 59, 61, 63, 69, 112, 114, 116–118, 121, 127, 129, 133

Bamberg Surgery Fragments, 110
Bernard of Gordon, 69, 120, 126
Barnuncus of Parma, 118
Bertinus de Rabis of Parma, xvii, 69, 118
Bladder stone, 75
Bologna, xviii
Bone, blood supply, 105
Bone fragment, penetrating brain, 63
Bonetus Locatellus of Bergamo, 133, 135
Brain and membranes, separation of, 73
Brain, blood supply, 113
Brainstem, 3
Bruno da Longoburgo of Padua, xiii, 69, 117–118, 125, 127
Bull dung, 21

Cabot, John, xvi
Callus, bony, 59, 61, 83, 97, 114
Cartilage, 7
Cautery, 47, 115, 124
De Cavilhao, Piedro, xvi
Cellula logistica, 116
Cellula memorialis, 116
Cellula phantasica, 116
Celsus, A. Cornelius, 118, 119, 126
Cerdo, Gera, 53
Cerebral compression, 57
  concussion, 65, 87
  contusion, 59
  edema, 115
  incision, 67
  laceration, 57, 63, 115
Cerebrospinal fistula, 116
Cerebrum, 3, 85, 97, 105
Circle of Willis, 116
Clonus, 126
Cogitation, localization, 67
Cold humor, 43
Conduction, bone, 114
Confusion, 107
Constantine the African, 42, 120
Contra coup injury, 118
Contracture of limb, 48
Coronal commissure, 3, 67
"Cracked pot sign", 126
Cranioplasty, 128
Cranium, 85
Crepitation, 33
Crown trepan, 123–124
Cupping, 73, 83, 119
Cupping bowl, 125
Cupping glass, 128

Debridement, 59, 77, 79
Delirium, 107

Dinus Florentinus, 46
Diploë, 103, 127
Drain, surgical, 47, 112
Dura mater, 59, 63, 103, 105, 113, 121

Elevation, bone fragments, 77
Elevation, depressed bone fragments, 93, 95
Elevator, 112, 122–123
Empiric sect, 69
Epilepsy, 67, 85, 109–110
Epilepsy, posttraumatic, 116, 125
Erasistratus, 117
Eschar, 63

Fees, 55, 101, 110
Fever, 59, 63, 67, 107
Florigerus, 69
"Four Masters", 44, 47, 114–115, 118, 120–121, 124–125, 127
Francis of Pedmont, 69, 117
Fungus cerebri, 115–116

Galea, 99, 103
Galen, ix, xxi, 5, 13, 27, 29, 41–46, 65, 67, 69, 79, 101, 114–117, 120, 121, 124, 126, 127
Gangrene, 114
Geleatius de Sancta Sophia, 53
Gentile da Foligno, 42
Gerard of Cremona, xvii
Glue, white, 11
Gout, 17, 19
Granulation tissue, 81, 83, 125
Guido, 127
Guidonus Faba, 69, 118
Guy de Chauliac, ix, xv, 44–46, 48, 110, 112–116, 118, 121, 124–125, 128, 131, 133, 135

Head injuries, closed, 118
Head wounds, 97
Head wounds, open, 89
Hemostasis, 124
Hippocratic writers, xxi, 45, 69, 109–110, 117–118, 120–121, 125–127
Hugh of Siena, xx
Hugo, 112
Hugo de Luca, 46
Humors, 5, 13, 29, 43, 57, 59, 65, 99, 103, 112, 121, 125
Hydrocephalus, 110

Imagination, cerebral localization, 67
Inflammation, 65
Injury, motor, 44
Instruments, surgical, 47, 53, 73, 77, 79, 81, 83, 111–112, 119, 121–125, 128
Intracranial pressure, 127
Irrationality, 67
Isaac Judaeus, 110

Jacme d'Aragramont, 126
Jiddah, xvi
Joannes de Vigo, 46
John of Gaddesden, 126
Joint pain, 23
  neurogenic, 21

Laceration, scalp, 59
Lancet, 123
Lanfranc, xv, 69, 117
Lenticular, 111, 123
Leonard of Bertapaglia, ix, x, xiii–xiv, xvii–xxi, 41–48, 109–121, 123–133, 135–136
Ligament, 7
Ligatures, 124
Lisfranc, 46, 109, 112, 116, 118, 121, 125
Loss of appetite, 107

Malgaigne, Joseph-François, 124
Mallet, 123
Mandible, 75, 103
Maxilla, 103
Mecca, xv–xvi, 51
Medulla, 73
Membrane, 7
Memory, 113
Memory, cerebral localization, 67

Meninges, 71, 113
  laceration, 113
Meningitis, 59, 107
Mirac, 45
Mochlia, 124
Modiolus, 123–124
Moicula, 77, 81, 112, 121, 123–124
Mondino de Luzzi, 45, 114
Montagnana, Bartolomeo, xviii
Moon, 73
Motion, voluntary and involuntary, 41
Musical instrument string, 101

Natural spirit, 117
Nerve, 7
Nerve attrition, 47
  attrition and torsion, 29, 33
  compression, 19
  constriction, 47
  contrition, 23
  corruption, 35
  debilitation, 21
  digital injury, 47
  fissures, 5
  fistulae, 5
  function, separation of motor and sensory, 37
  incision, 17, 21
  induration, 5, 35, 37, 39, 47–48
  injuries, 3–39
  injury, symptoms of, 3
  laceration, 5, 7, 11
  puncture, 5, 9, 11, 13, 15, 17
  sheath, 27
  stretching, 21
  suturing, 46
  torsion, 31, 35, 37, 39, 47–48
  transection, 5
  wounds, 9, 27
Nicolaus the Barber, 53
Nicolaus Physicus, 41, 43, 45, 116
Nigredo, 114, 129
Nucha, 42

Orbit, erythema, 113
Octavianus Scotus, 133, 135
Obtundation, 113

Padua, xiv, xvi–xx, 51, 67, 116, 129, 135
Paralysis, 3, 5, 23
Paralytics, 17, 19
Paré, Ambroise, ix
Paul of Aegina, 47, 119, 124
Perforator, 123
Pericranium, 113
Periosteum, 103
Peripheral nerve, 126
Peter of Albano, 93, 117, 120
Petrus de Argellata, 46, 69, 117, 127
Phlebotomy, 11, 19, 27, 29, 73, 112
Phlegmon, 27
Philagrius, 117
Pia mater, 59, 113
Pneuma, 117
Portal vein, 117
Psychosurgery, 110
Pulse, 75, 107, 121
Pus, 5, 9, 27, 31, 33, 48, 55, 57, 59, 61, 65, 99, 103, 112
Putrefaction, 13

Reason, 113
Renaldus de Villanova, 67, 69
Restlessness, 107
Rete mirabilis, 116–117
Rhazes, 42, 109
Rhodes, xvi
Riccardian Library (Florence), 129
Roger, xv
Roger of Parma, 117
Roger of Salerno, 69, 118, 120, 127
Roland of Parma, xiii
Rome, 51
Rugine, 123
Ruptorium, 81
Rupture, 33

Salerno Anatomy Dissection, 41
Sanies, 48, 114
Scalp laceration, 99
Scar tissue, 83
Separator, 122
Serapion, 69, 118
Sinew, 7

Singultus, 67
Siphac, 45, 113
Skull, anatomy of, 111–112
Skull fracture, 51–107, 110
  causes, 69–71
  comminuted, 59
  depressed, 95, 112–113, 123
  diagnosis, 95, 101, 126–127
  linear, 105
  non-comminuted, 61
  plicated, 71
Skull, inner table, 103
  middle table, 105
  perforation of, 69
  sutures of, 113
Sleep, 75, 121
Soranus of Ephesus, 120
Spasm, 3, 5, 9, 23, 63, 67
  facial, 15
St. Gregory of Nyssa, 119
Stomach, 97
Stuellis, 47
Stupe, 77
Submeningeal space, 127
Suture-ligature of blood vessels, xxiii
Sympathy, 97–99
Syncope, 67

Teeth, 101, 103
Tenta, 47
Terebelus, 123
Tetanus, 23–25
Theodoric of Cervia, xiii, 43, 46, 48, 69, 109–110, 112, 117, 129, 131
Thessaly, sect of, 117
Toothache, 103
Tremor, 23, 37
Trepan, 79, 121–123
  crown, 123–124
Trepanation, 110, 125
Trumpet in diagnosis of skull fracture, 101

Unnaturals, 57
Urinalysis, 75, 121

Varthema, Lodovico, xvi
Venice, 51
Ventricle, lateral, 115
Ventricles, cerebral, 67, 116
Ventricular tap, 110
Verona, 51
Vesalius, Andreas, ix, 42
Vital spirit, 117
Vomiting, 67, 107, 113

Wakefulness, 107
William of Salicet, xiii, 69, 112, 118
William of Verignana, 69, 117
Wine, 57, 97, 99
Withering of muscle, 35